Making Plant Medicine

Fourth Edition

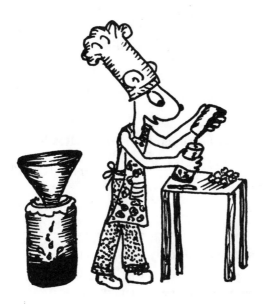

Disclaimer

Although all cultures on earth use plant-derived medicaments, we cannot recommend self-medication with plant products. Rather, we offer medicinal information in the context of historical usage and from personal experience, augmented by our studies of current research. Please seek the care and advice of a qualified healthcare practitioner for all medical problems. We have endeavored to provide responsible and specific cautions and contraindications for the herbs and preparations described in this book. However, be advised that iatrogenic,* idiosyncratic, and/or allergic reactions can occur, albeit rarely, regardless of the cautions employed. We do not accept responsibility for the use or misuse of any of the herbal information found in this book, or for any accident or injury caused by growing, handling, or ingesting plants or from attempting to follow processes described in this book.

*Definition of iatrogenic: physician-induced or imagined ailments.

—Richard A. "Richo" Cech and Herbal Reads LLC

Book orders may be directed to: Herbal Reads LLC
PO Box 26
Williams, OR 97544-0026
USA

www.herbalreads.com

Making Plant Medicine by Richo Cech

Cover art: Ann Gunter
Illustrations: Sena Cech

10 9 8 7 6 5

ISBN 0-9700312-3-8

Making Plant Medicine
Fourth Edition

by Richo Cech
illustrated by Sena Cech

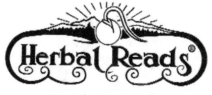

Herbal Reads
Williams, Oregon
2016

Table of Contents

Part 1

Part 2 – A Gardener's Herbal Formulary 103

TABLE OF CONTENTS

Appendices

Acknowledgements

Thanks to my most excellent family. You have accompanied me on this herbal path, always with love, patience, and trust—even when I gave you experimental tinctures and then stood there expectantly, waiting for the reaction! My wife Mayche thoroughly edited this fourth edition, making it more coherent and beautiful. This edition has been augmented by the addition of 28 new herbs in the formulary, a decade-long herbal sojourn that involved growing, extracting, and using an entirely new array of plants. This effort bolstered my faith in herbal remedies. It was a fantastic journey! We encourage gardeners to continue to grow diversity and welcome the medicine maker to convert this green energy into medicine for the people. This gentle art, which is perhaps as healing to the gardener and the medicine maker as it is to the person who takes the medicine, is a tradition rooted in our ancestry—as strong as an oak, as delicate as a violet.

Thanks to all my gardening friends. By growing these plants in your gardens and preparing them in this time-honored manner, you are keeping essential herbal traditions alive and well. If even one life is saved (and I've been told that at least one life *has* been saved) by knowing the herbs and preparations illuminated in this book, then I feel that all the effort given to researching, testing, and writing has been well-spent.

Our family welcomes you to this expanded fourth edition of "Making Plant Medicine." We love the earth and pray that all people love the earth and learn to love each other.

Richo

*This book is dedicated to my wife Mayche,
who has given the world three precious gifts:
Nadja, Jebran, and Sena.*

Part 1

Chapter 1
Granny and the Lunar Eclipse

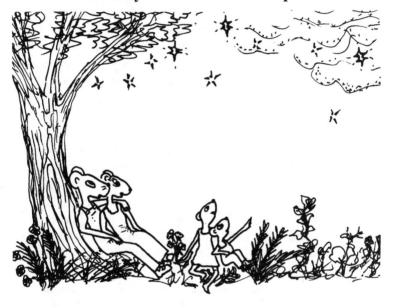

We sat cross-legged on the hillside, looking out over the dark valley. A summer wind moved through the thin stand of firs and alders. Mayche shifted closer to me, leaning on my arm. Moonlight sifted over the ridge before us, illuminating from beneath a few clouds that skittered by. Behind us loomed a huge rotten log, largely melted into red duff and crowned on its entire length by huckleberry bushes, which were now shadows in the dark. That morning, Nadja and Jeb had amused themselves by scrambling all over the log, putting one huckleberry after another into their chubby faces. To their taste, unjaded by candy or processed food, huckleberries were the best thing going. Our children reminded me of bear cubs, crawling fearlessly around in the tangled brush of these wild Oregon coast mountains. They slept like bear cubs, too, there in our laps. It was the night of a complete lunar eclipse, and we wanted to be there for it. But the full moon was loath to rise above the ridgetops and shine down into our narrow valley. We waited, and although the moonlight grew more intense and the crickets tuned up their serenade in anticipation of its coming, still the orb would not break clear. Then the moonlight from behind the ridge began to fade, and we realized that the eclipse was occurring out of our line of sight. We hunkered even closer and listened. The crickets hesitated, grated out a few more shrill notes, and then grew quiet. From far below, the waters of Elk Creek, unabated, tinkled and chimed over carven granite. The stars shone out over the still landscape, and the entire world forgot to breathe. Wordless, we waited for the moonlight to return, which it did quite slowly, much to the relief of the crickets, who soon got back to their music. We felt our way back down the rough, fern clad slope to our cabin. We would tuck the children into their pallet on the floor, check to make sure Granny was quiet in her bed, and finally slide under the covers to catch a few hours of rest before the dawn. But we never did go to sleep that night, because when we checked on Granny, she was dead. She'd slipped out during the eclipse, marking the end of her good life, and the end of a chapter in ours.

Bringing Granny out of the nursing home in Portland down to the farm was all Mayche's doing. It was a move opposed by the majority of the extended family, but not by Granny herself. Prior to the series of strokes that robbed her of her mental faculties, she had gotten out the Oregon map and penned a line, red and shaky, running from the metropolitan north down to the wilds of Elk City. Rumor had it that she told the relatives, "I know where I can go to get a square meal." It wasn't much to go on, but the map was a piece of hard evidence demonstrating Granny's desire to come live with us, and it was enough for Mayche. Her main opposition came from Uncle Ken, bless his heart, who believed that "managed care" was the way to go and had overseen Granny's removal to the nursing home. Mayche moved into Granny's comfortable house on 64th street, along with Ken, who was staying behind to take care of the estate. Nadja and Jeb were Mayche's allies in grinding away at his patience, assisted by her calculated purchase of large metal toy tops, the kind you get spinning by pushing down on a plunger on the top, which worked admirably well on the hardwood floors. As the tops vibrated across the polished floors with the wild kids from the woods scooting after them, tops and kids occasionally careening off the walls, Ken gritted his teeth, swirled the ice in his scotch, changed his mind, and relented to the move. He should've known better than to oppose the iron will of a pioneer woman.

Meanwhile, the situation at the nursing home was growing grim. Apparently the strokes had freed up a side of Granny that had never been let loose during her long, mundane life. The woman who had never once shouted, never allowed her husband to use an expletive more descriptive than "doggone," the woman who kept a miniature pond in the backyard and fed the goldfish daily, calling them to the surface with a sweet voice saying, "Fishy, fishy, fishy," was now using sailor's language in the nursing home. It was a complete personality overturn. Rumor had it that she was heavily tranquilized. In between bouts of drugged sleep, her poor broken record of a mind would make her call out to her sister who was not there. "Agnes" she would call, then, "Aaagnes! . . . Aaaagnes, please!" Over and over it would go, with nary a pause or variation. Or, she would get stuck on "Old McDonald had a Farm," starting at the beginning and singing in a trembling voice all the way up to "E I E I O," except for some reason the "O" just wouldn't come out. After hours and hours of "E I, E I, E I, E I . . ." even the managed care workers, who were supposed to be tolerant of this sort of thing, were ready for the loony bin. Everything, even Granny's choice of songs, was pointing to the farm.

During the several weeks Mayche stayed in Portland, I hurriedly finished construction on the north side of our cabin. The room, originally intended to accommodate our growing family, was now fixed up in anticipation of Granny's arrival, complete with insulated walls, baseboard heaters, and ramps for her wheelchair. I drove "Big Red," the firewood truck, up to Portland, reunited with my small family, and paid my respects to all the relatives, including Uncle Ken. He remained stoic in defeat, but his eyes evidenced a deep tiredness, along with at least a glimmer of relief. Mayche's dad helped me load all of Granny's necessities onto the back of the flatbed, and we tied everything down with hoses from the backyard. The goldfish were going to get mighty lonely.

Granny was convinced into the front seat of Mayche's car, and we followed the wobbly red line down south to the farm. Several nice pillows blew out of my truck on the freeway, but in our urgent need to get home, we did not even stop, but forged on. We arrived at the front gate in the late afternoon and crawled in low gear up the hill to a final halt in front of the cabin. The goats, which had free reign of the entire driveway and yard, stood in a group, probably awaiting their chance to jump on the hood of the car. But Nadja and Jeb shot out of the backseat and anchored the leaders with huge hugs around their necks. The goats watched in wonderment as we worked Granny into her wheelchair and across the pea gravel and mud, Mayche pulling at the front of the ungainly, poorly adapted apparatus, I pushing from behind. We breathed a sigh of relief when we finally hit the smooth boards of the ramp and pushed her into her new home.

There ensued a period of relative peace for Granny. She sat in front of a large picture window overlooking the hillside, where she could watch the play of the summer wind in the alder trees. She still spent long hours calling out "Agnes, Aaagnes, Aaagnes, please!" but the urgency and anxiety were falling from her voice. There were even moments when her mind arose out of the deeps like a fish going for a termite, and she registered a lucid glimpse of her surroundings. For instance, one day our black-and-white goat named Clover walked by the window, probably hoping to get a nip of nasturtiums from the window box. Granny said, "I saw a deer out there. If I'd-a had a gun, I would-a shot it!" One day she amazed us by getting up on her own and shuffling across the room with her walker, intent on examining some papers on the dresser. "There's a letter here from your sister, Edie," she told Mayche, rustling through the envelopes. Actually, there wasn't, but the fact that she correctly identified the familial relationship of two of her grandchildren, coupled with the self-reliant exploration, was hailed as a great success. Nadja and Jeb spent some time with Granny, too. When the kid goats were born, they were brought onto the porch for feeding. The children helped Granny hold a bottle while the baby goats jerked and sucked. Under the pure influence of the children's piping voices, their natural, unconcerned acceptance and compassion, and further influenced by the magnetic attraction and energy of the baby goats, Granny's furrowed brow finally gave way to a pure smile.

We had taken her off the tranquilizers right away and begged the closest naturopath to drive the eighteen miles on gravel roads to come and see her. He prescribed tincture of valerian, which we administered by the teaspoonful. Granny would grimace at the taste, but it gave her some needed rest, sometimes in bed, sometimes in the wheelchair, her gray head fallen forward on her ample bosom. The heavy, pervasive smell of valerian still reminds me of her.

This was actually our first experience with valerian, and it led us to investigate the plant further. I obtained some seeds from a now-defunct source and planted them in a flat in our greenhouse. They sprouted, and the seedlings sat in the flat for the entire summer, eventually going quite dry. I thought they had died of neglect, but midwinter came and a leak developed in the roof, dropping rainwater slowly down onto the flat. The dormant roots took off, magically filling the flat with vigorous, deeply divided leaves. I transplanted them out to the garden in the early spring, and by late spring we had shoulder-high, white-and-pink flowers that dipped in the breeze, the center of intense activity from diverse populations of gnats and other tiny pollinators. The smell, unlike the tincture, was delightful and intoxicating. I flipped through the pages of "A Modern Herbal," by Maude Grieve, and the names of the herbs attracted me. "What is this arnica?" I would ask myself. "And elecampane, it would be amazing to grow some of that." Concurrently, we began to identify the wild herbs that grew all around. Self-heal bloomed in profusion in the short, moist grasses of the orchard, and the entire family would go out and pull the heady blossoms, putting them in the shade on screens to dry. We made morning tea of the fresh flowers, and we used the dry flowers to make a medicinal tea for treating canker sores. The pain would go away and, in short order, the canker sores would also disappear. Since we liked the plant so much, we transplanted it into the vegetable garden and heaped some rotted goat manure compost around it. What had been a diminutive little creeper suddenly became a major floral statement in our garden, raising its head well above the bushy strawberries planted nearby and putting out hundreds of decorative cob-like flowers, intensely purple. This was the beginning of a long learning involving teas, extracts, and the domestication of wild medicinal plants.

Of course, Granny ate what we ate. She had been right about getting a square meal, but we were sure she hadn't bet on brown rice and tofu. We hoped that the improved nutrition would help her recover, but in actuality she was eating less and less. Mayche made attempts to get the old woman to wake up from the bad dream that seemed to have such a tight clasp on her mind and her spirit, and food was always a likely subject of conversation. Granny came from pioneer stock, and she had been justifiably proud of her cooking. One day, sitting before her with a plate of rather heavy whole-wheat waffles, Mayche forked up a bite for her. The old woman chewed and chewed. Mayche ventured to ask, "Do you remember how you taught me to make waffles, and we'd have them every Sunday for breakfast?" Granny got a glimmer of recognition in her eye and, having resolutely swallowed, answered, "Yes, but I wish I'd taught whoever made these!"

* * * * * * *

My goal in writing this medicine making book and formulary is to share the healing ways that have become a way of life for my family. I have endeavored to give people a complete and reasonable guide to understanding the simplicities and the intricacies of making herbal extracts. My recommendations are based on my experiences as a global wanderer and village herbalist and upon my long association with the physics of herbal extraction. My choice of herbs, formulas, and extraction techniques are the result of my experience as a gardener of herbs and as a student of Western herbalism. I am the first to admit that there are many other good and effective ways to use the herbs, and I do not pretend to have produced an all-encompassing document. I do believe that the herbs themselves will reveal their appropriate uses to the gardener. A sensitive relationship with the growing plant, coupled with the knowledge of good ways to harvest, process, and extract, will maximize the healing and minimize any potential to cause harm. Each herb is an individual, and each lends itself better to certain kinds of preparations, which can, in turn, be fine-tuned to the situation at hand, taking into account the constitution of the patient. In reviewing my own writing, I was a bit surprised by the duplicity of some of my recommendations. For instance, this is how you make an extract without measuring ingredients, and then this is why it makes sense to measure ingredients. But in thinking about it, I realized this to be a microcosm of herbalism: plants, people, and using herbs for health—the entire interconnected web—can be as simple or as complex as you find it. And even when approaching herbs with a mind toward simplicity, deeper understanding will inevitably ensue, leading to unforeseen levels of intricacy and intimacy. Sometimes the herbs work as the result of careful and purposeful application, while other times the mode of their healing can only be attributed to the workings of a great mystery that is beyond our calculated comprehension.

I believe that the herbs grown by our own hands in local gardens provide the strongest medicine we can possibly make and dispense to heal. I have repeatedly experienced the value of maintaining a relationship with the medicine from the time the seed is dropped into the soil to the time the extract is filtered. When I take this medicine or give it to my family and friends, I know exactly what plant it is, where it came from, how the extract was made, and what I want it to do. I have an unshakeable faith in the medicine, and this provides a strong foundation for healing. Since the beginning, the garden has been a haven of good values, both physical and spiritual. The act of gardening provides a balm for every wound. May your medicine be of the garden, and may it be of benefit to all.

Chapter 2
Making a Tincture
Basic Processes and Terminology

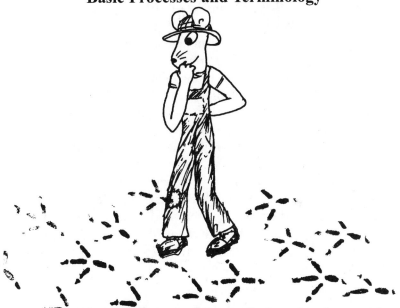

Early morning in the fallows of winter found me out in the middle of the garden, picking my way between the resting beds of roots and weeds, searching for signs of emerging life, of which there were scant few. I was taking a break from writing, renewing my brain and body with oxygen, and hoping for inspiration. Crows watched me from the oak tree in the nearby horse pasture, crows stark against the dim sky, blacker than the bare branches of the oak and as still as the clinging clots of mistletoe that also called that tree home. "No wonder crows are used for divination," I was thinking. "They are constantly observing the movements of men." My guess was they knew more about my habits than just about any other creature. Even if they didn't have the power to predict absolutely when I would be dumping the compost bucket, spreading cover crop seed, turning over the soil, or planting corn, they at least had the patience to wait for these activities, knowing that food would eventually happen. "Well," I thought, bending over to examine a tiny emerging seedling, apparently valerian, "if you crows are waiting for me to spread some more cover crop seed, you will have a pretty long wait." I noticed that the cornstalks were almost completely fallen and that the few ears rejected or forgotten during harvest had been stripped of their protective husks and picked clean to the cob. The crows would be getting hungry. I guessed that gnawing hunger was the down side for an animal that preferred to conserve energy rather than work to find food. So I made my rounds, admittedly wishing for spring, trying to make my mind be as still and watchful as the crows. But I kept imagining what it would be like to convince a crow to dip its feet in black ink and then walk across white paper or smooth white rocks. This would make something like writing, like dancing stick figures, hieroglyphics, or the pictographs that sometimes haunted my dreams. Still thinking about crow's feet, I returned to the seed house to work on the book about making medicines. I was hoping that my readers would find my writing more decipherable than the haphazard track of a crow and that they would gain an understanding of making tinctures, a process involving the twin, crow-like disciplines of activity and patience.

Terms

Tincture making has its own language—an unavoidable and necessary set of technical, obscure, and often antiquated words. Knowing these words is an initiation into the art of making medicinal extracts. Herbalism has its roots in a long history of extract making, and using this traditional language of extraction puts us all on common ground.

Tincturing: This is the process of making an herbal extract by steeping ground herb in a liquid menstruum, thereby infusing the liquid with the active constituents of the herb. These active constituents are sometimes known as "extractives." The tincture itself is the finished product, a relatively stable solution of extractives that is preserved (usually with alcohol) against deterioration.

Herb: An herb is simply a plant—an annual, biennial, or perennial— which is planted or voluntarily emerges in the spring and dies back down again in the fall. But when used by herbalists, "the herb" is an ambiguous term referring to a medicinal plant, or the fresh or dried plant material used for making a medicinal preparation. Although this name may call up an image of the fresh or dried *green portions* of a plant, it is also a loosely defined catchall term for *any part* of the plant, even the root, used in herbal therapy.

Menstruum: Sometimes known as the "solvent," the menstruum is the liquid portion of the tincture, usually consisting of a measured quantity of alcohol and water. The menstruum is always mixed in a clean vessel and then poured on top of the herb in the macerating container. When tincturing according to formula, the menstruum will not necessarily cover over the herb, but when tincturing the "easy" way, the menstruum is simply added until it covers the herb. Alcohol is used both because it is an excellent solvent for a wide range of constituents and because it preserves the extract. Water is used because it, too, is an excellent solvent for medicinal compounds. Some constituents are largely alcohol-soluble, while others are mainly water-soluble, and many herbs contain complex combinations of water- and alcohol-soluble constituents. As a consequence, the formula for each herb must take into account the kinds of constituents residing in the herb and their solubility, so that the finished tincture retains the activity of the herb and tastes like the herb itself.

Grinding: Sometimes known as "comminution," this is the process where the fresh or dried herb is reduced in size to create more surface area of extraction. Fresh herbs are finely minced with a knife or ground to a pulp in a blender along with the menstruum. The herb-menstruum slurry should "vortex" (i.e. swirl around, forming a tiny tornado in the center of the mass) inside the blender, resulting in a homogeneous product. Dried herbs are preferably stored in the whole form and reduced to a coarse powder by rubbing through a screen or by grinding in an electric coffee grinder, hammer mill, or blender just prior to tincturing. The optimum dry particle size is approximately that of coarsely ground cornmeal. If the grind is too coarse, the menstruum cannot sufficiently contact the cell structure of the herb in order to extract the active constituents. If ground to a fine powder, the herb will tend to pack inside the macerating container, thereby disallowing sufficient flow of liquids around the particles, again compromising the extraction of active constituents from the herb.

Macerating container: This is preferably a glass container with a wide mouth and a tight-fitting, corrosion-free, leakproof lid. The purpose of this container is to hold the macerating extract until it is time for pressing. Containers made of food-grade, high-density polyethylene (HDPE) are acceptable for maceration of most herbs, as are stainless steel vessels. However, if the herb contains essential oils (e.g. anise, rosemary, or hyssop) then the tincture is best macerated and stored in glass.

Macerating extract: This is a name for the slurry of herb and menstruum during the process of maceration. In many cases the fresh herb pureed with menstruum looks a little like volcanic magma, and it is just as slow as molten rock to pour from the vessel into the pressing cloth.

Maceration: This is the process of steeping the ground herb in the menstruum for a period of (usually) three weeks, sufficient time for the liquid portion to become thoroughly saturated with extractives from the herb. Maceration is usually best accomplished at room temperature in a dark place, such as a cupboard.

Shaking: Sometimes known as "succussion," this is the process where the macerating extract is thoroughly shaken in the macerating container to allow for complete contact between the menstruum and the herb. The container is grasped in both hands and vigorously agitated until the contents are thoroughly remixed. Shaking is not particularly important in making fresh herb tinctures, where the process of extraction is basically dehydration of the plant cell by alcohol. However, in dry herb extraction, the process of shaking is quite essential, because over time the dry herbs can clump at the bottom of the container, and agitation puts the herbal particles back into intimate contact with the solvent.

Labeling and record-keeping: Label all macerating containers and finished tinctures with the name of the herb and the date of tincturing. This is the minimum labeling required to keep track of what you are doing. For those who would like to take this one step further, here is a run-down of good manufacturing practices, which will allow you to keep better track of several tincturing runs without confusion. First, the macerating containers must be properly labeled with the common and Latin name of the herb and the starting date, which is the date when the herb and men-struum were first combined. This label, or an exact copy of it, will accompany the extract through all phases of maceration, pressing, settling, and filtering, in order to ensure the identity of the end product. Second, keep a tincturing logbook where you record all relevant details about the identity and source of the herb and the making of each tincture. This includes the dates, the formula, the weights and volumes of all components, the final volume yield, and special notes. This logbook will help you maintain consistency from one tincture to the next, keep track of any significant details that might help improve future tinctures, or perhaps elucidate the cause of the rare disaster that can occur. Third, give a consecutive lot number to each extraction run, recording this number both in your logbook and on your bottled tinctures. This will allow for full recall of all manufacturing details, including the irrefutable identity of the tincture, in order to avoid confusion or liability at a later date.

Pressing cloth: This is a multilayered piece of cheesecloth or a single layer of pressure-resistant polypropylene cloth designed for holding the macerating extract during pressing. Any suffi-ciently sized piece of fabric, such as linen, will also serve the purpose, but tensile strength is a necessary prerequisite. There is nothing quite so messy as cleaning up a "dandelion explosion" resulting from the failure of a pressing cloth under high pressure!

Pressing: This is the process wherein the macerating extract is thoroughly squeezed or "expressed," thereby separating the herb from the liquid, which is now infused with the activity of the herb. This can be accomplished by hand. Drape the pressing cloth over a bowl, pour the macerating extract into it, close up the top, and by kneading, squeezing, and twisting, wring as much liq-uid into the bowl as your strength will allow. This can also be accomplished with a tincture press. A tincture press is composed of two parallel platens on a frame that is rigged with a hydraulic jack and a pan fitted with a drain hole and a hose. The macerat-ing extract is poured into a pressing cloth inside the pan and the cloth is folded over the top of the mass of herb to prevent it from squeezing out the sides. Then the platens are jacked together, thereby efficiently forcing the liquid from the herb. Not only does this press out the menstruum, but it also forces the *intrinsic plant water* out of fresh plant material. The tincture flows from the pan down a hose and is captured in a receiving vessel. Using a tincture press greatly increases the yield from a given batch of extract, making the most of your expenditure for alcohol and your valuable work in growing the herbs.

Marc: The press-cake, composed of nearly dry plant fiber that has been divested of most of its medicinal virtue, is called "the marc." Removed from the wrinkled pressing cloth, broken up, and set outdoors in a pile layered with comfrey leaves, grass clippings, manure, or other nitrogen-rich materials, this marc makes about the best compost obtainable anywhere. In a few short weeks, if turned and allowed to heat up, it will become black dirt that can be recycled back to the garden as a nutrient-rich side-dressing for vegetable plants and medicinals.

Settling: The crude tincture, that is, the tincture which has been pressed but has not yet been filtered, is kept in the receiving vessel, securely capped, and left alone on a shelf where it is allowed to settle for a period of time. Overnight settling is usually sufficient. Any solid material that finds its way into the tincture through the porous pressing cloth or by dint of sloppy pressing will settle out on the bottom of the container. This material is known as "sediment" or the slightly more descriptive word "sludge." It is not in solution with the tincture and is best excluded before it starts to draw extractives out of solution (see "Precipitation" page 15).

Decanting through a filter: The clear, settled tincture needs to be filtered through multiple layers of clean cheesecloth, an unbleached coffee filter, or a coarse laboratory-grade filter paper. The filter is set up in a funnel resting in a receiving container. Take care not to make a tight seal between the funnel and the receiving container, in order to allow the escape of displaced air, lest the air attempt to escape back up through the filter and cause a blopping mess reminiscent of the bubbling paint pots of Yellowstone Park. The settled tincture is "decanted," that is, poured off from the top, the clear liquid slowly introduced into the filter without disturbing the sediment on the bottom of the jar.

Most clear tinctures will filter rapidly, so long as the sediment is not poured into the filter. By the way, thick, mucilaginous tinctures such as marshmallow or comfrey will *never* go through paper. These are customarily filtered through one or two layers of cheesecloth, which will exclude any chunks of herbal debris, while allowing the thick tincture to flow through.

Storage containers: The ideal storage container is a small-mouthed, amber glass bottle with a closely fitting lid. The finished extract is poured into this container and dispensed into smaller dropper bottles as needed. The tincture is stored at room temperature, out of direct sunlight. Properly made, an alcoholic tincture has an expected shelf-life of at least three years. Some herbs, such as goldenseal, contain antimicrobial compounds that assist in stabilizing the extract, making it last for decades. Others, such as valerian and shepherd's purse, must be tinctured anew each year, since they contain chemically unstable compounds that will rapidly degrade.

Precipitation: A tincture is a solution of soluble plant constituents in a solvent menstruum. The menstruum will hold these constituents in solution for a period of time—often years—depending on various factors. Poor filtration technique, exposure to light in storage, temperature change (especially from warm to cold), or chemical degradation of extractives can cause solid particles to "precipitate out" of the tincture. Such particles are known as "precipitates," and they usually settle out to form sediment on the bottom of the storage container. Regardless of whether precipitates are composed of active constituents or inert proteins, precipitation is an undesirable event. In order to limit the occurrence of precipitates, the tincture is best stored out of the light and at consistent room temperature. If precipitates form, the tincture can be refiltered in order to arrest the process, albeit temporarily, and then returned into a clean, dry storage container. Massive precipitation accompanied by a marked color change in the tincture, an "off" smell, or the apparent loss of characteristic taste or potency means that the tincture should be discarded and made anew with recent ingredients.

Chapter 3
Tincturing Made Easy

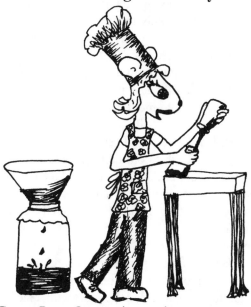

Grants Pass, Oregon is a retirement town, a place that draws true urban dwellers as a kind of all-American oasis, a little piece of mid-America on the west coast—not too far from relatives in Seattle or Los Angeles, but far enough away to not have to breathe the big city air. On a bright fall day I bounded, whistling, up the steps of the Jim Wood Insurance Agency and swung through the front door to stand in the center of the living room, suddenly feeling a little perplexed at the apparent change of furniture. A mousy-haired woman came out of the kitchen to see why her door was slamming. When she saw me, she nearly dropped her coffeepot. I said, "Hey, I'm really sorry. I thought I was in the insurance agency." She took my arm in a matronly grip, turned me around, and ushered me precipitously back outside, saying, "They're next door," and pointed to the nearly identical blue-gray frame house with the shingle outside reading, sure enough, "Jim Wood, Grange Insurance." With my tail tucked between my legs, I skulked over the lawn and tentatively opened the door. The customary scene put me back on track—the easy chairs were set around, and the usual certificates of completion

17

hung on the walls. I further anchored my reality by checking the familiar knickknacks on the mantelpiece that had evidently been set there new in the 50s, having now grown into antiques. I once determined that they had likely been dusted 2,607 times in their lives, at the rate of one dusting per week. The mind does funny things while waiting for insurance.

Valerie greeted me from her spreading desk, a pretty young lady with wavy blonde hair and a thin face. She was blessed with an impeccable memory and an indisputable understanding of procedure. Impossible to ruffle, Valerie was always friendly, but wielded the power of receptionist, as well as agent. She had good reason for this confidence, because the solid force of her father, Jim Wood, backed her up. He had a direct view of her desk area from his own office, a dark room off to the side, and knew everything that was going on. He delivered free-form comments at will, aimed at Valerie or the customers, whether they were there to see him or not. He sat in dominion before his desk, wearing a black leather vest that expanded mightily across his barrel chest. A huge, black plastic phone sat within easy reach. Despite his balding head, he ruled the roost with a face that never failed, even in humor, to command. Behind him and on the sides towered files recording every home, every car, every insurable bauble owned by his hundreds of customers, going back for generations. There was not a computer in sight.

I started to greet Valerie, but before we could get around to business, a voice erupted from the side room. "Hey!" said Jim. "Are they still lettin' you drive?" "Yep," I answered. "Have they let you out yet for your daily exercise?" And the banter went on like that, with Valerie waiting, tapping her pencil. She had bought some fresh echinacea roots from us a week or so previously, and I wanted to find out what had become of them.

Mayche had delivered the roots and described what to do. "Well," said Mayche, holding out one of the bristling roots as an example, "you have to wash it thoroughly, cut it up into small pieces, and put them in the blender. Then cover the pieces with some strong alcohol and blend for a few minutes until it gets mushy, and then pour it into a canning jar and put on the lid. You let it sit like that on a shelf for two or three weeks and you shake it every day. Then you pour it through cheesecloth or an old linen napkin and squeeze out the tincture into a bowl. You can store the tincture in a brown bottle. That's about it." Valerie took it all in. "Can I use vodka?" she asked. And Mayche replied, "Vodka is perfect."

"How's your echinacea doing?" I asked Valerie. But before she could answer, Jim was at it again. "She treats that thing like a baby!" he rumbled. "She's got it there in the back room, and she's all the time checkin' it, talkin' to it, and shakin' it. She thinks I don't know she's nippin' on that stuff!" "Oh Dad," said Valerie, "stuff it!" She turned to me with a wink. "I have to tell you," she said, "that was the hardest thing I ever tried to cut up. Worse than woody carrots. First I tried cutting it with a paring knife, and then I chopped it with a meat cleaver. I had pieces of roots all over the kitchen. I used a new toothbrush and scrubbed every piece. Then I nearly wrecked my blender. But I think it's good." She got up, retrieved the jar from the back room, and gave it to me for my approval. The blended roots did indeed look very clean, and the liquid, which just covered the fibrous mass of roots in the jar, was already taking on a bright amber color. I unscrewed the lid, being careful not to dump the whole thing on her desk full of papers, dipped in my finger, and took a taste. The familiar sensations speedily arose—the increased output of saliva and the numbing, buzzing sensation. I screwed back on the lid and turned toward the dark door of the inner office. "Jim," I said, "your daughter makes real good stuff!"

Easy Tinctures

Medicinal herb gardeners can readily make effective liquid extracts using only the simplest of tools—things found in every country kitchen: a sharp knife or pruning shears, a cutting board, canning jars with lids, cheesecloth, and a bowl. Grinders and blenders can speed the process, but they are not necessary. Making tinctures according to the specific formulas given later in this book requires the use of a gram scale, and a graduated cylinder for measuring liquids, but the simplified procedures described in this chapter require very little measuring and no weighing at all!

Procedure for making an easy tincture:

1) Chop the fresh herbs or grind up the dried herbs.
2) Place the herb in a glass jar, labeled with the current date and the name of the herb.
3) Add sufficient liquid menstruum to cover the herbs.
4) Screw on the lid, put the jar in a dark place at room temperature, and shake at least once daily.
5) After 2 or 3 weeks, pour the contents of the jar through several layers of cheesecloth and express the liquid.
6) Allow the liquid to settle in a clean jar overnight.
7) Decant the clear liquid through a filter paper.
8) Store in correctly labeled, amber glass bottles, out of the light.

Making Menstruum the Easy Way

I heartily recommend using grain alcohol (190 proof = 95% pure alcohol) to make the menstruum, if you can get it. The more you use, the "heartier" you get. But seriously, there is no better agent for the purpose, both by dint of its ability to extract a wide array of medicinal compounds from plants and because of its ability to preserve.

The best water to use in tincturing is distilled water. To the extent that water contains dissolved minerals or additives, the efficiency of extraction, or the "dissolving power" of the water, will be correspondingly lessened. If you cannot get distilled water, then use pure springwater or well water—not city water containing chlorine.

As a menstruum for *dry* herbs, make "diluted alcohol" by combining one part by volume of grain alcohol with one part by volume of distilled water. If grain alcohol is not available to you, then forget adding water and just use vodka or other spirits. The alcohol you use for dry tinctures must be at least 40 proof (20% pure alcohol) or you risk the possibility that the extract will not be adequately preserved.

As a menstruum for *fresh* herbs, use grain alcohol without adding water. If grain alcohol is not available to you, then just use the highest proof alcohol you can find. The alcohol you use for fresh tinctures must be at least 80 proof (40% pure alcohol), or you risk the possibility that your finished extract will not be preserved. Always choose spirits that do not contain a lot of flavoring additives. A tincture works best when it tastes like the herb, not some other flavoring agent that was in the alcohol to start with. Also, the grain alcohol can only "hold" a certain quantity of extractives, and if the manufacturer has added a flavoring, the content of active constituents will be correspondingly lower.

Harvesting and Processing Herbs for Tincturing

Fresh aerial parts: Harvest leaves and flowers of plants in the midmorning, after the dew has evaporated. Leaves generally contain the highest degree of medicinal activity just prior to flowering (e.g. sage). The leaves of biennials are usually harvested in the summer of the first year of growth (e.g. mullein). Flowers are harvested in the early stages of maturity, often in combination with associated immature buds and leaves (e.g. Saint John's wort). If the stems are succulent and contain the active principles of the plant (e.g. skullcap), then they can be left in the tincture. If they are very woody and/or do not carry the characteristic taste of the plant (e.g. catnip), then it is best to exclude them from the tincture.

To make the fresh herb tincture, put the leaves and/or flowers on a cutting board, and finely mince them with a sharp knife. The idea is to break through as much of the cell structure as possible, while increasing the surface area for extraction. Lightly pack the minced herb into a quart jar or other macerating vessel and cover completely with the menstruum, screw on the lid, then set the tincture aside to macerate.

Fresh roots: Roots are usually dug at the end of the growing season or during dormancy, when they have stored their energy for the winter. Wash them thoroughly, using clean water and a high-pressure hose, or scrub brush if necessary, to remove dirt and rocks that may be hiding in the crevices. Sometimes the crown must be split before washing in order to get the root as clean as possible. Use pruning shears to remove pieces of stem, old wood, or rotten portions. Place the clean roots on a cutting board and slice them into thin sections. Or, if they are very woody, use pruning shears. Diagonal cutting, as is typically employed in the preparation of Asian food, is a good practice. The idea is to make the pieces small enough so they can be easily ground up, or if they are to be tinctured in sliced form, to expose the inner cell structure of the root to the menstruum. Pack the fresh root pieces into the macerating jar, pour the menstruum over the root pieces until they are just covered with liquid, screw on the lid, then set the tincture aside to macerate.

Blender method: Blending the fresh, chopped plant or roots assures that the cell structure is thoroughly broken up. Put the coarsely minced herb or chopped roots in a blender and cover them with alcohol. Put on the lid. Turn on the blender, letting it grind the herb into homogeneous slurry. Once the herb vortexes in the blender, you can add a few more leaves or root pieces at a time through the hole in the lid of the blender, continuing for as long as the blender will accept the new input. When the blender can take no more pieces of herb, then it is time to stop blending. By the way, during this process take care not to get alcohol splashed in your eyes, and never, never stick your fingers into the blender while it is operating. If you have to dislodge stuck blades or manually stir the contents to promote vortexing, then remove the blender vessel from the base before proceeding and use the handle of a wooden spoon. Those blades are sharp! Pour the slurry into the macerating jar, cover, and set aside to macerate. This method produces a slightly stronger extract than the "chop-and-cover" methods previously described, largely because you can get more herbal material into the same amount of menstruum. However, if you do not have a mechanical press, it can be harder to get the tincture back out of the macerating extract during the pressing process. The best overall advice I can give is to use a blender if you have a mechanical press and to use the chop-and-cover method if you will be squeezing the tincture out by hand.

Dry aerial parts: Harvest leaves and flowers in the midmorning, after the dew has evaporated from the plants. It generally works best to dry the entire aerial parts of the plant (leaf, flower, and stem) by placing the herb on screens in a warm, dark, and airy location or by tying into bundles and hanging from open rafters. If using a heated, forced-air dehydrator, the thermostat is set at a low setting so that the temperature does not exceed 110° F (~38° C). The herbs are then turned several times to avoid "sweating" and to afford even drying. Once the plants are dry, you can further process them, working on a clean sheet or on a smooth table. Crush the leaves and flowers by hand and set them aside in a large bowl or a clean bucket. Sometimes it helps to rub the plants through a coarse (¼ inch = 0.64 cm) screen to further break up the leaves and flowers and exclude the stem material. The dried stems may be composted or tied up in bundles to use as an aromatic fire-starter in the winter. If you have a hammer mill, coffee grinder, or blender, you can grind the herb before proceeding. Otherwise, rub the dried herb through a ⅛ inch (0.32 cm) screen until it is reduced to a coarse powder.

Dry seeds: Harvest seeds when they are fully mature and easily separated from the plant. Seeds are best harvested in the afternoon of a very dry day. If the seed pours readily from the capsule (e.g. motherwort), simply turn the plant upside-down into a clean bucket and give it a shake. The seed will accrue in the bottom of the bucket. If the seed adheres to the stem (e.g. angelica), then rub the umbels between your hands, allowing the free seed to drop into the bucket. If the seed will not shake or rub from the plant (e.g. echinacea), then cut the seed heads, dry them in the shade, crush or coarsely grind them, and separate the seed from the chaff using screens or the wind. If there are spiders or other small insects helplessly reeling around in the newly harvested seed, then spread it out on a sheet in the grass and let them crawl away before gathering the seed up for further drying. Seed may be cured for a few hours in direct sun, as long as the temperature does not exceed 90° F (~32° C). The seed is laid out on pieces of sheets on top of screens and stirred several times to ensure even drying. Then the laden screens are suspended in a drying room or other open, airy location until the seed is thoroughly dry. Before tincturing, the seed is ground to a coarse powder or bruised by rubbing on a fine stainless steel screen.

Making the tincture of dry aerial parts or seeds: Pour the crushed or ground herb or seeds into the macerating vessel. Because the dry herb will absorb liquid and swell, only fill the macerating jar about halfway up with the herb. Slowly pour the menstruum on top of the herb until it is completely covered by liquid. Screw on the lid, shake, and allow to settle for an hour or two, and then check the jar again. If the herb has swollen above the surface of the liquid, add more menstruum until the herb is again inundated. Then, set the jar aside to macerate. By the way, it is interesting to note that dried herb swells much more substantially when the menstruum contains a lot of water, and it swells minimally when the menstruum contains mostly alcohol.

Dry roots: Dig the roots while the plant is dormant and wash them thoroughly. If you have no machinery for grinding the roots after they are dry, then you must make them into thin slices while they are fresh. Once dried, most whole roots are quite immutable, and require power machinery or a large hammer to powder them. Dehydrate the root pieces, out of the sun, on a screen in a warm, airy, and dry location. It usually takes a week or two for them to dry thoroughly, so that they snap when flexed. If you have a hammer mill, blender, or coffee grinder, you can then further reduce the dried root pieces into a coarse powder (about the consistency of coarsely ground cornmeal), which is optimal for extraction. Or, you can use the dried, sliced root pieces without further grinding.

Fill the macerating jar a little over half full with dried root powder or slices, and slowly pour the menstruum on top. Make sure the herb is thoroughly wetted. Keep pouring until the herb is covered with menstruum, then secure the lid, leave it to soak for an hour or two, then check the jar again. If the roots have swollen above the surface of the liquid, add more menstruum until they are again covered. Then shake and set aside to macerate.

Further Notes on Processing

Shaking and macerating: Shake your macerating tinctures at least once a day. This will ensure that the herbal particles are truly coming into contact with the menstruum. The tincture gets stronger over time. Optimal macerating time depends on the hardness of the materials being extracted. Fresh chamomile blossoms, blended, only take a few days to finish. Dried wild yam root, sliced and not powdered, could easily take two months to fully extract. Once the prescribed maceration time is over and the free liquid in the jar has taken on the color of the herb and tastes strongly like the herb, then you can proceed to pressing.

Pressing: Here is the hands-on (or hands-in) technique: A good pressing cloth can be made from several layers of clean cheesecloth or a single layer of clean linen draped over a large glass or ceramic bowl. Pour the macerating extract into the pressing cloth, gather the edges together, and squeeze. Collect the crude tincture in the bowl. If your macerating tincture was composed of minced or crushed herb or root slices, then this hand process will be pretty efficient. If you ground things up in a blender, and squeezing the mucilaginous, amoeboid mass in your hands produces only a disappointing drizzle of liquid, you may have to go looking for someone with a press.

Settling and filtering: Put the crude extract in a labeled jar and set it on a shelf, leaving it undisturbed overnight. Very turbid extracts may take longer than overnight to settle, but you will know that the settling is complete when the demarcation between the clear extract and the bottom sludge is well-defined. In the morning, slowly decant the liquid through a coffee filter or several layers of clean cheesecloth. Collect the finished tincture in a clean jar.

Storage: Store the finished tincture in an amber glass bottle, appropriately labeled and dated, in a cool place out of the sun. An empty wine or beer bottle, closed with a cork or rubber stopper, is an excellent storage vessel for larger quantities of tincture. Amber glass bottles with droppers are the preferred tool for administering drop dosages of liquid extracts. They can be purchased fairly inexpensively and reused.

* * * * * * *

The methods described in this chapter for making tinctures without weighing or fancy measuring give very satisfactory results, and you don't have to feel embarrassed if you opt to make extracts this way. The tinctures will be a bit variable in strength, as the process is not standardized. So this year's black cohosh extract may turn out a little different than last year's. If this doesn't bother you, it probably won't bother the person who is taking the extract, either.

Even with standard processing, where you weigh and measure all the ingredients, there will still be a little yearly variation in your tinctures. Plants are individuals, and they do not all have the same strength. Come to think of it, people are individuals, too. They do not all have the same strength, or the same sensitivity, either. Weak extracts may agree with some folks better and still do their work very effectively over time. Furthermore, weak extracts can be made to act strongly and quickly simply by increasing the dosage.

When "tincturing the easy way," you may actually end up producing extracts that are *weaker or stronger* than what are produced by following the recipes in the formulary section of this book. Using tinctures that are made according to formula provides a baseline of consistency. Otherwise, one may gain a feel for the strength of each batch by administering a moderate dosage to start, maintaining this dosage (if it works) or increasing the dosage according to the constitution of the patient and in response to the severity of the problem. You'll get the feel for it. The main thing is to keep in mind that this is medicine—make it with good heart and dispense it in good faith.

Chapter 4
Extracting Order from Chaos
The Mathematics of Tincturing

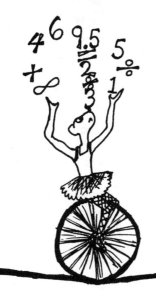

Why would one want to go through all the trouble of measuring ingredients and tincturing according to standard formulas if the tinctures could be made by the methods described in "Tincturing Made Easy?" Well, there are reasons. In making tinctures, when you mix together the herb and the menstruum, it is encouraging and efficient when the proportions come out right the first time according to expectations. In using tinctures, it helps to know from batch to batch, and from year to year, that your tinctures are made in a consistent manner. Take this story, for example.

Uncle Harry, who is actually not as hairy on top as you remember, comes to visit for a suspiciously unspecified period of time, stopping by on his way back from spending three months on the beach in Hawaii eating papayas. Unfortunately, he brings with him a nasty staph[1] infection of the leg, an aftereffect of intimate contact with a piece of ragged coral, an incident he

---

[1]A gram-positive bacterial infection characterized by redness and swelling.

describes in shifting detail, a story involving big waves and a three-legged sea turtle. Uncle Harry has bad associations with doctors and, despite your plea for him to see a professional, seems more content to lie on the couch in your living room and watch his leg rot than to get on down to the emergency room of the local hospital. You, of course, would like to see him get better, not only because you like Harry, but also because if he does not get better, he may never leave.

You get out the burdock, dandelion, echinacea, and Oregon grape tinctures, mix them together as an "antistaph brew," pour them into a 2-ounce dropper bottle, and tell Harry to take 1 dropperful 5 times a day without fail and drink water like it is going out of style. Harry puts down his fashion magazine and gratefully starts to "dose up," dropping the tincture into a little water in a cup as he props himself on a slightly scabby elbow, there on the couch. You pray that the herbs will do their work. That night, you have trouble getting to sleep, worrying that the herbs may not be strong enough to cure the infection. Wondering if you should have told him to take 2 droppersful 5 times a day instead of just 1, you finally drift off.

Luckily, the next day Harry's condition is stable and, after three days, his leg is much, much better. He is now off his couch, singing in the kitchen, and concocting a "smoothie" of orange juice and bananas. He does not wipe the counter or rinse the blender and he leaves the empty glass on the rug next to the couch. You go shopping.

The day after that he wakes up really frisky, dancing in his socks outside the bathroom door. You take this opportunity to let him know that today is cleaning day and you would like the ceilings dusted, all the back windows done, and, by the way, does he know how to fix lawn mowers? Within the hour, he is in the front hall, bags in hand, whistling his way out the door. "It's been nice, but I gotta run . . ." He goes out.

Pressing your palms against the inside of the door, you breathe a gigantic sigh of relief, then gaze ruefully at your partially collapsed couch cushions. Emerging from this reverie, you walk over to your desk, take out the "herbs" notebook, and record this bit of herbal information: "Equal amounts burdock, dandelion, echinacea, and Oregon grape; 1 dropperful, 5 times a day—successfully treated staph infection in leg. Thank goodness!"

Cleaning day abandoned, you go take a bath, swirling a lavender pillow around in the hot water with your left foot, leaning back, eyes half closed, mentally dancing with Harry's three-legged turtle . . .

Now the next year, you make the same tinctures and, as usual, you don't measure the ingredients. The opportunity arises again to use the "antistaph brew," and you are glad to make some up. The neighbor's 10-year-old, Jason, shows signs of impetigo[2] and his mother would rather not run him through the medical mill. Jason weighs in at about half as much as Harry, so you figure 15 drops (a half dropperful) of the tincture 5 times a day will be a good starting dosage. That night your mind keeps you awake again, this time with the nagging suspicion that this year's tinctures might be less strong than what you made last year. (When it comes right down to it, you can't know how strong an extract is unless you measure the ingredients.)

After two days, you find that Jason is really not responding very well to the therapy. Despite his mother's innate distrust of any medicine stronger than homeopathic arnica, she takes him in to the emergency room and, of course, the doctors put him on penicillin immediately. You wish he had been able to overcome this problem by stimulating his own immune response and by fighting the infection with herbs, avoiding the potential side effects of penicillin. Was his failure to respond to the herbs because the tinctures weren't as strong as last year, or are there other contributing factors? Does Jason surreptitiously consume large quantities of illicit candy bars? If so, this could easily subvert herbal therapy. You suspect this may be the case, remembering his bad teeth and flashing on the one time that you gave him a ride and he produced two candy wrappers in twelve minutes, one of which was left stuck to the upholstery of the back seat. But you can't be certain of why he failed to respond. You resolve to measure the ingredients next time you make tinctures, thereby removing at least one of the variables from the whole picture.

---

[2]An acute, contagious bacterial skin disorder characterized by pustules.

* * * * * * *

Processing your own good herbs in a consistent manner will make you trust your medicine all the more, because it takes some of the guesswork out of making tinctures and also takes the guesswork out of dosage recommendations. Following find a concise explanation of the standard ratios and formulas involved in making fresh and dry tinctures, conventions which can be used to assure optimal extraction, full preservation and relative consistency of strength of your tinctures. We will also look at the absolute alcohol content of various kinds of spirits, in order to assure your ability to mix a menstruum of the correct alcohol content. Using this information, you will be able to make the best possible tinctures, in accordance with the solubility of the various constituents found in the herbs. Specifically, we will examine ways to convert grain alcohol and other alcoholic spirits into the most commonly used menstruum, "diluted alcohol." We will also examine the mathematics involved in determining the efficiency of any given extraction, that is how much finished tincture you end up with in relation to how much total liquid went into the formula. Finally, we will look at how to determine the water content of fresh herbs, enabling you to calculate the finished alcohol content of tinctures, thereby assuring adequate preservation.

Standard Tincturing Ratios
1:5 (50A:50W)

The formula for making a tincture according to standardized proportions consists of 2 important ratios, as in the example above. Following find a discussion of these 2 ratios.

Herb:Menstruum ratio: This is the first ratio in a given formula, seen above as 1:5. It compares the weight of the herb (either fresh or dried) to the volume of the total liquid menstruum. Weight is expressed in grams (g) while volume is expressed in milliliters (ml). Thus, a typical dry tincture might read 1:5 (1 part in g of dried herb combined with 5 parts in ml of menstruum to make the extract) and a typical fresh tincture might read 1:2 (1 part in g of fresh herb combined with 2 parts in ml of menstruum to make the extract). For example, 100 g of dried motherwort leaf and flower would be combined with 500 ml of menstruum to make a dry plant tincture. Or, 100 g of fresh chamomile flowers would be combined with 200 ml of menstruum to make a fresh plant tincture. So, this first ratio is basically a manufacturing standard, which simply tells you how many parts of plant material are added to how many parts of liquid in order to make the tincture.

Alcohol:Water ratio: This is the second ratio, representing the proportions of the various liquids that are combined to make up the menstruum. For instance, the basic menstruum for a dry herb consists of 50% grain alcohol combined with 50% distilled water. This menstruum would be expressed as (50A:50W) as in the opening example. This menstruum is also known as "diluted alcohol."

The second ratio may get more complicated if ingredients other than water and alcohol are used. For instance, a menstruum containing glycerin might look like this: (50A:40W:10Gly), where the menstruum consists of 50% alcohol, 40% water and 10% vegetable glycerin.

Or, the second ratio may be simpler if only alcohol is being used, as is often the practice with fresh herbs containing largely alcohol-soluble constituents. In this case, the menstrum would look like this: (100A), where the menstrum consists of 100% alcohol.

Alcohol[3]

Grain alcohol: This is pharmaceutical grade alcohol made from grains (usually corn)—not petroleum products. Through the liquor store, it is available under the brand names of "Everclear" and "Clear Spring." Grain alcohol consists of 95% pure alcohol (absolute alcohol) and 5% water and contains no flavoring additives. These, along with the organic options following, are the easiest and best substances to use for herbal extraction, due to their edibility and efficacy as solvents. Grain alcohol preserves the tincture when the volume of grain alcohol measures at or above 22% of the total liquid volume.

3The molecular formula for alcohol is C_2H_5OH.

Organically certified 95% pure alcohol: Distilleries offer superior products made of non-gmo, organically certified corn, sugar cane, grape, and wheat. The wheat alcohol is the most neutral in taste and may be found as a certified gluten-free product.

Other kinds of alcohol: If grain alcohol is not available, then you must use weaker spirits. Choose the one with the highest "proof" and the least flavoring additives. If you are using weaker spirits, such as vodka or rum, and you still want to be able to mix a menstruum with a specified alcohol content, then you will have to compensate. You will have to determine the absolute alcohol content of your chosen spirits and add the correct amount of water to produce the desired menstruum. Following find the steps and equations required to produce diluted alcohol with any given spirits. First, look on the label of your chosen alcoholic beverage and find the "proof." It will read something like "120 proof," or perhaps "80 proof."

Formula to determine the absolute alcohol content of spirits:

P = proof of spirits
C = absolute alcohol content of the spirits

$$\frac{P}{2} = C$$

Example 1: Grain alcohol is 190 proof, so to determine the absolute alcohol content of grain alcohol:

$$\frac{190}{2} = 95$$ [95% absolute alcohol content in grain alcohol]
(The remaining 5% is water.)

Example 2: To calculate the absolute alcohol content of 120 proof rum:

$$\frac{120}{2} = 60$$ [60% absolute alcohol content in rum]
(The remaining 40% is water and flavoring.)

Diluted alcohol: This is useful stuff, because it is the main menstruum called for in extraction of most dried herbs. It is really easy to make if you have grain alcohol, using the formula (50A:50W). You simply combine equal volumes of grain alcohol and distilled water. Diluted alcohol contains 47.5% absolute alcohol and technically is only made from grain alcohol. 100 proof vodka contains 50% absolute alcohol and is free of flavoring agents, so for all practical purposes this is the best substitute for diluted alcohol made with grain alcohol. If you do not have grain alcohol or vodka, you can come up with a reason-able facsimile using other highly alcoholic spirits (higher than 100 proof), such as 120 proof rum.

Formula to make menstruum of a specified absolute alcohol content from highly alcoholic spirits other than grain alcohol:

D = desired % of absolute alcohol in menstruum
C = absolute alcohol content of spirits
S = % of spirits used in making the menstruum

$$\frac{D}{C} \times 100 = S$$

Example: To make diluted alcohol from rum, which has an absolute alcohol content of 60%, you need to dilute the rum down to 47.5% absolute alcohol content by the addition of a little water.

$$\frac{47.5}{60} \times 100 = 79 \quad \text{[79\%[4] of total menstruum is rum]}$$
$$\text{(The remainder will be water.)}$$

---

[4]In this book, the final figure of each equation is rounded. Percentages are rounded to the nearest percentage point, volumes to the nearest ml, and weights to the nearest gram. For the purpose of home medicine making, a fraction of a percentage point, ml, or g are insignificant units of measure.

To determine how much water to add to the rum to make diluted alcohol, subtract the 79% from 100%.

100 - 79 = 21 [21% of water added to make diluted alcohol]

So, if you wanted to mix up 1000 ml of diluted alcohol using this kind of rum, you would combine 790 ml of rum (79% of total) with 210 ml of distilled water (21% of total), yielding 1000 ml of menstruum at the desired 47.5% absolute alcohol content.

Determining the Absolute Alcohol Content of Fresh Plant Tinctures

Fresh plants contain between 40% and 90% water, depending on how their tissues are made and how much water they received during their growth cycle. If you are making a fresh plant tincture and you want to know the absolute alcohol content of the finished product, then you must account for the water that was contributed to the tincture by the plant.

There are 2 reasons why it is important to know the percent of alcohol in a finished tincture:

1) Optimal extraction of active constituents from herbs is dependent on their greater or lesser solubility in water and in alcohol. This issue is thoroughly discussed in Chapter 5, in "Solubility Factors," pages 46–8

2) A tincture is not fully preserved unless the absolute alcohol content measures above 20%. This is very easy to determine in dry herb extraction, but is a little more complicated in fresh herb extraction. All the formulas for fresh plant tinctures given in the formulary section of this book are designed to account for the water content of the fresh plant, resulting in fully preserved tinctures. However, if you are designing your own formulas for herbs *not* covered in this book (or other reliable formularies), then it makes sense to take a drying sample and to do the math to make absolutely certain that your extract is preserved.

Drying sample: To determine the water content of a plant, take a sample of the fresh, undried plant and weigh it. A convenient quantity is 100 g fresh weight. Place the sample on a screen in an herb dryer or next to the wood stove. It usually takes between

2 and 3 days to dry the sample. Horsetail dries overnight, while mullein leaf may take weeks. Once the stems "snap" when you break them and the flower or leaf material "crinkles" when you crush it, then the sample is truly dry, and it is time to weigh it again. If you are unsure whether or not it is dry, weigh it and dry it some more. If the weight does not change, it is dry. The difference between the original weight and the dry weight is equivalent to the amount of water in the sample. Conveniently, the specific gravity of water is 1, so every gram of water is also equivalent to 1 ml of water.

Formula for determining the water content of a fresh herb sample:

F = weight of fresh herb
D = weight of dried herb
W = water content of the herb in % of total fresh herb weight

$$\frac{D}{F} \times 100 = \% \text{ dry weight}$$

100 - % dry weight = W

Example: Fresh hyssop herb weighing 100 g was dried down to 30 g dry weight. To figure the proportion of dry weight:

$$\frac{30}{100} \times 100 = 30 \quad [30\% \text{ dry weight}]$$

100 - 30 = 70 [70% water content in the herb]

If made into a fresh extract, the 100 g of hyssop herb would thus contribute 70% of its weight, which is equivalent to 70 ml of water, to the tincture.

To figure plant water in ml, multiply the total fresh herb weight by the percentage water content of the herb:

100 x .70 = 70 [70 ml plant water in tincture]

Tracking the Efficiency of Extraction

Given the intrinsic value of herbs as well as their monetary cost and the value of the human labor in growing and processing them, it is good to be able to track the efficiency of extraction in order to help maximize the tincture yield. The efficiency of extraction is best expressed as a "percent return" figure. In order to arrive at this figure, you compare the actual volume yield of the tincture with the total liquid volume.

Volume Yield: This is the actual final measured volume of the filtered tincture. The finished tincture is a composite of all the liquid contributed by the fresh herb in addition to the menstruum, minus any evaporation, spillage, or moisture remaining in the marc, pressing cloth, or filter paper.

Total Liquid: This is the sum of the liquid menstruum plus the calculated water content of the entire quantity of fresh herb used in the tincture.

% Return: This figure represents the efficiency of extraction by comparing the total liquid to the volume yield.

Formula for figuring % return:

Y = volume yield
L = total liquid
R = % return

$$\frac{Y}{L} \times 100 = R$$

Example: Fresh hyssop herb tincture made at 1:2 (100A).
You are making a tincture of fresh hyssop herb. The herb weighs 5,550 g. You now add the appropriate amount of grain alcohol according to the formula:

5,550 x 2 = 11,100 [11,100 ml grain alcohol needed]

We have already determined that the hyssop contained 70% plant water, so the calculated water content of the entire quantity of fresh herb used in the tincture is 5,550 x 70%:

5,550 x .70 = 3,885 [3,885 ml plant water in tincture]

Therefore, the total liquid available to the tincture was:

11,100 + 3,885 = 14,985 [14,985 ml total liquid in tincture]

After pressing and filtering, the actual volume of the finished tincture was measured at 13,200 ml.

$$\frac{13,200}{14,985} \text{ x } 100 = 88 \quad [88\% \text{ return}]$$

So, we can say that the process was basically 88% efficient in reclaiming the total liquid input to the tincture.

A return of 90% is very good, and generally means that you have a good press. A return of 70% is not very good and may generally be attributed to poor pressing efficiency. Very woody herbs (e.g. Oregon grape root) tend to retain liquid, thereby resulting in lower yields, whereas very soft, leafy herbs (e.g. chickweed) give up their liquid more easily under pressure and generally result in higher volume yields.

Absolute Alcohol Content

Formula to figure the absolute alcohol content (i.e. the content of pure alcohol) of a finished tincture:

M = absolute alcohol content of the menstruum
L = total liquid
T = absolute alcohol content of the tincture.

$$\frac{M}{L} \times 100 = T$$

Example: For your same fresh hyssop tincture you already know that the total liquid is 14,985 ml. Now you need to figure the absolute alcohol content of the menstruum. Since the menstruum consists of grain alcohol (which contains 95% absolute alcohol), the calculated alcohol content for the entire quantity of menstruum is:

11,100 x .95 = 10,545 [10,545 ml absolute alcohol in menstruum]

To figure the absolute alcohol content of the fresh hyssop tincture:

$$\frac{10,545}{14,985} \times 100 = 70 \quad \text{[70\% absolute alcohol content in tincture]}$$

      Figuring the absolute alcohol content of a fresh herb tincture that is extracted with a menstruum containing alcohol *and* water is a bit more complicated. This will be covered in Chapter 5, in "Basic Formula for Fresh Herb Tinctures," page 41–2.

* * * * * * *

38

Employing mathematics during extraction will improve the consistency of your final product, but it should be understood that your math can only be as reliable as your laboratory technique.

Practices that will make your mathematically derived alcohol content match the actual alcohol content of the finished tincture are:

1) Zeroing the scale before starting.
2) Weighing accurately.
3) Reading the level of liquid (the meniscus) in a graduated cylinder from the *side*. Reading from the *top* results in "error of parallax."
4) Avoiding spills, great and small.
5) Keeping lids on all containers in order to limit evaporation.

However, even given the most careful laboratory technique, the actual alcohol content of the finished product will be altered to a certain extent by the herb itself. Besides contributing water, herbs also contribute nonwater extractives to the solution that we call the tincture. Alcohol will dissolve alkaloids, fats, fixed oils, essential oils, glycosides, resins, sesquiterpenes, wax, etc. out of the cell structure of the herbs, and these will, to a certain extent, contribute to the final volume of the extract. Water will dissolve alkaloids, gums, polysaccharides, proteins, saponins, tannins, etc. from the herb. These also will contribute to the final volume of the tincture. Depending on the volume taken up by these extractives (which is usually almost negligible), this may or may not significantly affect the calculated absolute alcohol content of the finished tincture. A clear example of the influence of plant extractives on the final yield, and therefore also on the alcohol content of the extract, is tincture of gumweed (*Grindelia* spp.), which gives consistently high yields due to the presence of large amounts of alcohol-soluble resins.

Chapter 5
Tinctures: Basic Formulas, Solubility Factors, and Dosage

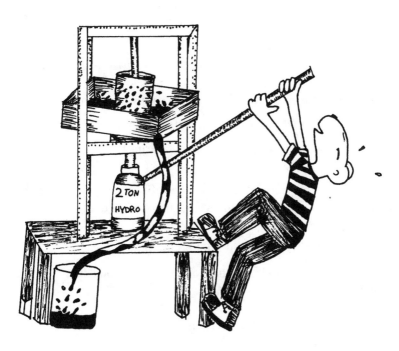

Basic Formula for Fresh Herb Tinctures
1:2 (75A:25W)

The ratios shown above represent the best all-around formula for making fresh herb tinctures. If you are trying to make a tincture out of a fresh herb that is not listed in the formulary of this book, use the ratios above as your default formula. This section gives a step-by-step procedure for how to make a good tincture from fresh herbs using this formula. Specific examples are given, showing how an actual tincture would be put together. The headings (e.g. formula, herb weight, menstruum, plant water content, yield, percent return, and alcohol content) are applicable to any fresh tincturing process, and form the basis for accurate record keeping.

Example 1: Skullcap (tincture of fresh flowering aerial parts)

Formula: 1:2 (75A:25W)

Fresh herb weight: 300 g (total weight of herb used)

Menstruum: 600 ml (total volume of liquid added to the herb, composed of: 450 ml grain alcohol + 150 ml water)

Plant water content: 73%
To figure the plant water content in the tincture, multiply the fresh herb weight by the percentage of plant water in the fresh herb (determined by running a drying sample; see pages 34–5).

300 x .73 = 219 [219 ml plant water in tincture]

Yield: 750 ml (measured yield after filtering)

% return: 92%
To figure the percent return (the efficiency of the pressing process), add the volume of the menstruum to the volume of the plant water.

600 + 219 = 819 [819 ml total liquid in tincture]

Then divide the yield by the volume of the total liquid in the tincture and multiply by 100.

$$\frac{750}{819} \textbf{ x 100 = 92} \quad [92\% \text{ return}]$$

Absolute alcohol content of finished tincture: 52%
To figure the absolute alcohol content of the finished tincture, first multiply the volume of grain alcohol by .95. This gives the volume of absolute alcohol used in making the tincture.

450 x .95 = 428 [428 ml absolute alcohol]

Then divide this volume of absolute alcohol by the total liquid and multiply by 100 to give the absolute alcohol content as a percentage. This how one determines the absolute alcohol content of a fresh herb tincture made with a menstruum containing both alcohol and water.

$$\frac{428}{819} \textbf{ x 100 = 52} \quad [52\% \text{ absolute alcohol content in tincture}]$$

Example 2: Echinacea (tincture of fresh 2- or 3-year-old dormant roots)

Formula: 1:2 (75A:25W)
Fresh root weight: 500 g
Menstruum: 1000 ml (composed of: 750 ml grain alcohol + 250 ml water)
Plant water content: 70% (350 ml plant water in tincture)
Yield: 1,215 ml
% return: 90%
Absolute alcohol content of finished tincture: 53%

General procedure for making fresh herb tinctures:

1) Coarsely chop and weigh the fresh herb or root and put it in a blender.
2) Measure and mix the menstruum in a separate jar.
3) Pour the menstruum over the herb and blend thoroughly.
4) Pour the blended slurry into a macerating container.
5) Cover tightly, shake, and set to macerate in a dark place at room temperature. Label with date and herb name.
6) Shake daily for a period of 2 weeks.
7) At the end of this time, pour the macerating herb into a pressing cloth and express thoroughly by hand or with a tincture press.
8) Collect the crude tincture in a jar, label, and set it on a shelf to settle overnight.
9) The following morning, decant the clear liquid through a filter and collect the finished tincture in a jar.
10) Store in labeled amber glass bottles, well-stoppered, in a cool room, and out of the sunlight.

Depending on the total amount of fresh herb being used and the capacity of the blender, the entire quantity of fresh herb may need to be processed in several or many blendersful. It is often desirable to start the blender with the full measure of menstruum and only a little herb or a few root pieces, gradually adding the pre-weighed herb, a few pieces at a time, through the hole in the lid of the blender, while the blender is running. Do not ever put your fingers in the blender! As each blenderful is completed, it can be poured into a large macerating jar, the whole mixed together, and then macerated as a single batch.

Example of a typical blenderful: 150 g: 300 ml. At a 1:2 concentration, it was determined that the ideal amount of herb to fill the blender one time was 150 g of fresh herb combined with 300 ml of liquid.

Basic Formula for Dry Herb Tinctures
1:5 (50A:50W)

The ratios shown above represent the best all-around formula for making dry herb tinctures. If you are trying to make a tincture out of a dried herb that is not listed in the formulary of this book, use the ratios above as your default formula. This section gives a step-by-step procedure designed to give a full overview of how to make a good tincture from dried herbs. Specific examples are given, showing how an actual tincture would be put together, with weights and volumes of ingredients, final yields, etc. The headings given (e.g. formula, herb weight, menstruum, yield, and alcohol content) are applicable to any dry tincturing process, and form the basis for accurate record keeping.

Example 1: Motherwort (tincture of dried leaves and flowers without the stems)

Formula: 1:5 (50A:50W)
Dry herb weight: 150 g (total weight of herb used to make the tincture)
Menstruum: 750 ml (composed of: 375 ml grain alcohol + 375 ml water)
Yield: 670 ml (measured yield after filtering)
% Return: 89% (the efficiency of the pressing process)
Absolute alcohol content of finished tincture: 48%
The absolute alcohol content of a dry herb tincture is equivalent to the absolute alcohol content of its menstruum.

Note: The entire batch fit in a quart jar. Larger batches would have to be made using larger macerating containers or be macerated in several vessels, each containing herb and menstruum in proportion according to formula.

Example 2: Ashwagandha (tincture of dried roots of dormant 1- or 2-year-old plants)

Formula: 1:5 (50A:50W)
Herb weight: 200 g
Menstruum: 1000 ml diluted alcohol (composed of: 500 ml grain alcohol + 500 ml water)
Yield: 820 ml
% Return: 82%
Absolute alcohol content of finished tincture: 48%

Coverage: When tincturing according to formula, you may find that a dry, fluffy, ground up herb like motherwort is barely wetted by the menstruum. The liquid will not cover over the herb. Do not be tempted to add more liquid, as this would result in a dilute tincture. Macerate and press out the wetted herb in the usual manner, thereby producing a finished tincture of dependable strength and consistency.

General procedure for making dry herb tinctures:

1) Grind the dried herb down to the consistency of coarse cornmeal by using a suitable mill or, if applicable, by crushing the herb and rubbing it through a screen.
2) Measure and mix the menstruum in a separate jar.
3) Weigh the herb and pour it into the macerating container.
4) Slowly pour the menstruum over the ground herb.
5) Cover tightly, shake, and set to macerate in a dark place at room temperature. Label with the current date and herb name.
6) Shake daily for a period of 3 weeks.
7) At the end of this time, pour the macerating herb into a pressing cloth and express thoroughly, either by hand or by using a tincture press.
8) Collect the crude tincture in a jar, label, and set it on a shelf to settle overnight.
9) The following morning, decant the clear liquid through a filter and collect the finished tincture in a jar.
10) Store in labeled amber glass bottles, well-stoppered, in a cool room, and out of the sunlight.

Solubility Factors

Here is a listing of some of the important classes of medicinal compounds found in herbs, along with their general solubility in the primary edible solvents used in herbal pharmacy. As long as the constituent profile of the herb is well-understood, this information can assist the herbal medicine maker in choosing the menstruum that is most appropriate for drawing out the active constituents from the herb. This is especially helpful if the preferred menstruum for extracting the herb is not already listed in this book or in other reliable formularies. The ultimate goal is to design the menstruum so that the extract tastes like the herb and carries the same balanced effect as the herb. For example, by looking at this list it will be clear that marshmallow, which contains water-soluble mucilage as its main active constituent, is best extracted with a menstruum containing primarily water. Conversely, gumweed, which owes most of its activity to the presence of resins, is best extracted with a menstruum containing primarily alcohol. A more chemically diverse herb such as goldenrod, which contains water-soluble tannins and saponins, as well as alcohol-soluble essential oils, would best be extracted with a menstruum containing equal parts of alcohol and water.

Class: Alkaloids

Herb examples: bloodroot, goldenseal, lobelia, ma-huang, and motherwort

Activity: Each alkaloid tends to have a very specific action, but viewed as a class, the activities of the alkaloidal herbs are extremely diverse, including effects such as: anticancer, antiseptic, antispasmodic, emmenagogue, expectorant, galactagogue, nervine, stimulant, etc.

Solubility: Alkaloids are very soluble in alcohol and only slightly soluble in water. In extracting alkaloidal herbs, acidification of the menstruum with apple cider vinegar sometimes increases the potency of the tincture (see "Chapter 6, Vinegar Extracts"). Alkaloids are sometimes rendered unstable by heating, and alkaloids are also sometimes neutralized by tannins.

Class: Essential Oils (Volatile Oils)

Herb Examples: anise, eucalyptus, hyssop, lavender, peppermint, sage, and thyme

Activity: Herbs containing essential oils will exhibit activities such as: antiseptic, anti-inflammatory, expectorant, hypotensive, insect repellent, sedative, etc.

Solubility: Essential oils are very soluble in alcohol and generally soluble in cold-pressed fixed oils such as olive oil, sweet almond oil, or jojoba oil. Essential oils are only slightly soluble in water and grudgingly soluble in glycerin. Using heat in the processes of drying, cooking, or extraction of these herbs will result in the volatilization of essential oils and loss of efficacy.

Class: Glycosides

Herb examples: gentian, hawthorn, rhubarb, licorice, and milk thistle

Activity: Herbs containing glycosides can exhibit activities such as: analgesic, antioxidant, bitter, cardiotonic, laxative, etc.

Solubility: Glycosides are usually soluble in both alcohol and water.

Class: Mucilage (Gums)

Herb examples: comfrey, elecampane, flaxseed, marshmallow, mullein flowers, purslane, and slippery elm

Activity: Mucilaginous herbs are emollient to the mucous membranes and soothing to injured tissues. Herbs in this class tend to be high in nutritional content and immune-stimulating.

Solubility: Mucilage is strictly water-soluble and is precipitated out of solution by the addition of alcohol. Mucilage is also better extracted with cold water than with hot water. Therefore, mucilaginous herbs are best made into cold infusions, not hot teas, and are tinctured using only sufficient alcohol to preserve.

Class: Polysaccharides

Herb examples: astragalus, boneset, burdock, dang-shen, and echinacea

Activity: Herbs containing medicinally active polysaccharides are generally immune-enhancing and nutritive.

Solubility: Polysaccharides are water-soluble and precipitated out of solution by alcohol.

Class: Resins

Herb examples: calendula, gumweed, and rosemary
Activity: Resins often provide effects such as: expectorant, relaxing, counterirritant, stimulating, antispasmodic, bitter, etc.
Solubility: Resins are soluble in alcohol and hot oil, but insoluble in water.

Class: Saponins

Herb examples: American ginseng, American wild yam, chickweed, figwort, mullein flowers, violets, etc.
Activity: The effects of herbs containing saponins are very diverse, including: adaptogenic, diuretic, expectorant, anti-spasmodic, etc.
Solubility: Saponins are water-soluble.

Class: Tannins

Herb examples: self-heal, tea, and witch hazel
Activity: Tannins precipitate soluble protein. They may also render certain alkaloids inactive. Herbs containing tannins are generally antiseptic, astringent, and styptic. They are often used to ease pain, reduce swelling and bleeding, and to speed healing of wounds.
Solubility: Tannins are soluble in water, alcohol, and glycerin. Tannins in solution are bound up and rendered inactive by the addition of milk.

* * * * * * *

Although in medicine making and in herbal therapy it is helpful to know the constituent makeup of the various herbs, this knowledge should not be an invitation to oversimplification or reductionism. In other words, you still need to know the herb itself, not just its chemistry, in order to be able to derive full benefit from it. Herbs work best as whole entities, not as isolated compounds, because the constituents contained in herbs often work together to create a whole effect. Furthermore, the herbs themselves have an innate nature that is larger than their chemistry. In much the same way that humans cannot be defined by their elemental makeup, medicinal herbs cannot adequately be defined by their constituent profile. When we take the right herbs for a given condition, the body is naturally guided back to a healthy and balanced state. The result of this purposeful interaction between plants and humans is perhaps less a matter of chemistry than a commingling of interdependent souls.

Dosage of Tinctures

The advantages of taking herbs in tincture form are many. Tinctures are stable, convenient, and due to the fact that they are cold-processed and preserved from enzymatic change through the addition of alcohol, they probably represent the actual chemistry of the herb more closely than any other preparation. Because they are liquid, the dosage can be regulated almost infinitely, from near-homeopathic dosages (1 drop diluted in water and taken over time) to heroic dosages (¼ ounce or more taken over the space of a few hours).

Tinctures are quickly and readily absorbed into the bloodstream through the lining of the stomach and, because of this, their effects are not dependent upon the efficiency of digestion. This is an advantage over solid preparations (tablets or capsules), but it also means that one must remember to take the tincture several times daily in order to sustain the effect. Absorption is a bit more efficient if the extract is taken between meals, and tasting the herbs without the buffering of other food will maximize the benefits, because in many cases, especially with bitter or immune-enhancing herbs, the taste is part of the effect. The most important time to remember to take the extract is just before bed. At this time the body is in its most receptive phase, allowing the herbs to tonify the body organs and orchestrate the body processes in a clear and uncomplicated manner.

The basic dosage recommendations given in this section apply to tinctures that are safe for general consumption. Please check the formulary section of this book for potential contraindications. The decision to take an herb should be based on good herbalism and the advice of a qualified health care provider.

Dosage for infants (10 weeks to 3 years): The average dosage for infants is 2 to 5 drops well-diluted in water, milk, or juice, taken 3 to 5 times daily. Most herbs are safe for consumption by infants, but low-dose botanicals (e.g. arnica, lobelia) should be avoided. Infants are very sensitive to herbal therapy and should be given the minimum effective dosage. In treating infant colic, it often makes sense for the mother to take the herb, delivering the influence to the child by way of the breast milk.

Dosage for children (4 years to 10 years): The average dosage for children is 5 to 15 drops well-diluted in water or juice, taken 3 to 5 times daily. As with infants, the low-dose botanicals should be avoided in favor of gentler herbs.

Adult dosage: The normal adult dosage of most tinctures is 30 to 60 drops (1 to 2 standard droppersful) diluted in a little water and taken 3 to 5 times daily. This represents a therapeutic level of intake, and is an appropriate starting dosage.

Senior dosage: Seniors tend to be very sensitive to herbal therapy. A good starting dosage is 1 dropperful (30 drops) taken 3 to 5 times daily.

The remainder of this chapter consists of an overview of variables that will influence these basic dosage recommendations.

Body weight: Small individuals with high metabolic rate require smaller doses. Larger individuals with slow metabolism require larger doses. For example, a little woman who has eaten nothing but bread and jam all day, flitting about the library from book to book like a hummingbird after nectar, will probably notice the effects of a fairly small beginning dosage of tincture. The logger slumped down in an easy chair in the corner of the library reading the paper (automotive section—used 4x4s), who has made the bulk of his daily caloric intake out of cans of "beanie weenies," will require a larger dose of medicinal herbs to notice any effect.

Severity of the condition: Acute phase conditions may call for more frequent dosage, while certain chronic conditions may require less frequent dosage. For instance, at the beginning phase of an acute infection, echinacea tincture is taken with frequency, as often as every ½-hour for maximum effect. Conversely, the tendency toward chronic upper respiratory infection may be suitably addressed by taking astragalus only once or twice daily as a tonic. In most cases, one will begin to feel an effect from the herbs after 2 or 3 doses, and the size and frequency of the dose can be regulated in accordance with the degree of effect desired.

Nature of the herbs: Certain herbs (e.g. milk thistle) can be taken several times daily for as many days as one desires, without experiencing any deleterious effects. Other herbs (e.g. comfrey) contain potentially toxic substances. These should be taken only at recommended dosage and only for a short period of time. Low-dose botanicals (e.g. arnica) that contain very active constituents are listed in the formulary section of this book, along with the recommended maximum dosages.

Frequency of dosage: Because herbs work gently, making changes by slowly nudging the body toward homeostasis, taking small amounts of tincture with regular frequency is the desired model. Large, single doses have less effect than smaller, frequent doses. Therefore, once the beginning dosage has been set according to body weight, it makes sense to increase the dosage by taking the herb more frequently—not by taking larger doses.

Appropriate use: It should go without saying that herbs have a physiological effect, and if used inappropriately, they will act adversely. For instance, it would not make sense for someone suffering from an inflamed liver to use a liver-stimulating herb like Oregon grape.

Pregnancy: Many herbs are not advised for use during pregnancy, generally because they may adversely affect the vascular system, the uterus, or the fetus. These herbs are identified in the formulary section of this book under the "Contraindications" heading.

Hypersensitivity and allergic responses to herbs: Although most herbs are safe for most people, there is always the potential for idiosyncratic reactions to occur. Over the years, I have seen a good number of these. For instance, although nettles is a good blood purifier and can help alleviate allergies, too many nettles taken too frequently can cause allergic dermatitis (urticaria). Certain individuals will be hypersensitive, and the reaction may occur even within the confines of the recommended dosage. If an individual is obviously sensitive (e.g. very young, very old, very thin) it is best to start with low dosage with an eye out for any adverse reactions, gradually increasing the dosage until the desired effect is realized.

An adverse reaction is sometimes thought to be a "proving" for the herb, meaning that the herb has somehow caused latent infirmities to be expressed. Practitioners ascribing to this idea sometimes recommend the continued use of the herb under question, perhaps at lower dosage or in homeopathic form. However, it is my opinion that uncomfortable reactions are a strong message to discontinue the use of that particular herb.

Drug-herb interactions: Herbal therapy and allopathic therapy make strange bedfellows, especially if the medical doctor is unaware that herbs are in the picture or if the herbalist is unaware that drugs are in the picture. Herbs can increase the effects of certain drugs. For instance, red clover thins the blood, and if taken along with the blood-thinning drug warfarin,[5] the result can be disastrous. On the other hand, certain herbs, such as blue flag, can alter the rate at which drugs are metabolized by the liver. Other herbs, such as marshmallow, can slow the rate of absorption of drugs into the bloodstream. Saint John's wort in particular is prone to interacting with and altering the activity of common pharmaceutical medications including oral contraceptives, antidepressants, and the heart medication digoxin. In short, whether you are in the care of an herbalist or a medical doctor, each needs to be made aware of which allopathic medicines, supplements, and herbs are being taken. This will help minimize adverse reactions.

---

[5]Warfarin is an anticoagulant agent that was originally invented to be used as a rat poison. However, it was soon discovered that small doses administered to humans act as a blood-thinner. The most common pharmaceutical drug of this type is called Coumadin.

Chapter 6
Vinegar Extracts

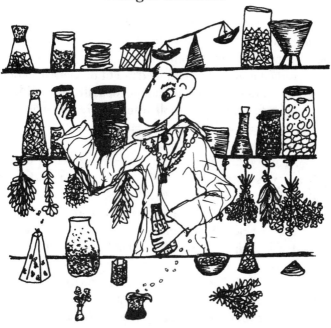

Before the invention of distilled alcohol, the typical menstruum used for making liquid extracts was water, vinegar, or wine. With the advent of distillation, higher proof alcohol, to a large extent, replaced these substances, due to its superior extraction and preservation capabilities. But simple vinegar, which has an acidity factor of 5%, lends its own unique qualities to an extract. It is a passable solvent and preservative and can be used as a pure menstruum in order to avoid the use of alcohol. When used in *combination* with alcohol, it will sometimes assist in the extraction of alkaloidal (base) substances from herbs. This is where its true pharmaceutical value lies. When an acid menstruum is poured over certain alkaloidal herbs, a reaction occurs wherein the alkaloids are turned into alkaloidal salts, which then become available to the solution.[6] A menstruum containing both alcohol and vinegar sometimes will render more active principles from an alkaloidal herb than can alcohol alone. Such an extract is known as an "acetous tincture."

In contrast, extracts containing 100% vinegar as a menstruum are called "aceta" (the singular is acetum). Aceta have a limited shelf-life and are not usually very potent in comparison to extracts containing alcohol. Furthermore, dry herb aceta are generally stronger than fresh herb aceta, which are really closer to salad dressings than tinctures. By the way, neither pure vinegar aceta nor acetous tinctures are "herbal vinegar," which is a term applied to fancy vinegar in a clear bottle, flavored by the addition of a few sprigs of fresh flowering herbs. Our goal in making more potent vinegar tinctures is for the vinegar to carry the properties of the herb at a therapeutic level.

Actually, organic apple cider vinegar (ACV) itself is a very healthful substance, as it is rich in potassium and enzymes. Including ACV in your diet, whether alone, on salads, or as a menstruum for herbs, will tend to improve digestion, thereby increasing resistance to most diseases. The commonly available "distilled white vinegar" which is made of diluted acetic acid does not, in-and-of-itself, deliver the same health-giving effects as true ACV, which is our preferred acidic menstruum. The one downfall of apple cider vinegar is that it is already somewhat "loaded" with extractives, so that it is not as efficient a solvent as one might hope. But nobody's perfect.

---

[6]This footnote supplied by Nadja Cech: "The reaction involves changing the alkaloids into alkaloid salts. The reason this works is that all alkaloids are organic bases having a nitrogen group that can become protonated (i.e. $R-NH_2$). The alkaloids in their basic (neutral) form aren't as soluble in polar solvents, such as water or alcohol, as the alkaloids in their protonated form (in which the $R-NH_2$ group becomes an $R-NH_3+$). This is why increasing the acidity of the solution helps with solubility. The alkaloids react with the acetic acid in the vinegar and become protonated and the polar solvent stabilizes the charges on the protonated alkaloids. The alkaloidal salts that form exist as dissociated anions and cations in solution and would only become associated with each other if you boiled off the solution. This would leave a crystalline residue consisting of the charged alkaloids and their counterions. In the case of acetic acid, the counter ion is acetate (CH_3COO-) so the alkaloid salts that would form would be $R-NH_3+COO-$. Here the alkaloid is the cation and the acetate is the anion."

Basic Formula for Dry Herb Aceta
1:7 (100ACV)

Example: Thyme dry herb acetum

Formula: 1:7 (100ACV)
Herb weight: 50 g
Menstruum: 350 ml apple cider vinegar
Yield: 300 ml (measured yield after pressing and filtering)
% Return: 86%

General procedure for dry herb aceta:

1) Grind the herb to a coarse powder, or crush it thoroughly by rubbing through a fine screen.
2) Weigh the herb and pour it into the macerating container.
3) Measure and slowly pour the vinegar over the herb.
4) Cover tightly, shake, and set to macerate in a dark place at room temperature. Label with current date and herb name.
5) Shake daily for a period of 2 weeks.
6) At the end of this time, pour the macerating extract into a pressing cloth and express thoroughly, either by hand or with a tincture press.
7) Collect the crude acetum in a jar and set it on a shelf to settle overnight.
8) The following morning, decant the clear liquid through a filter, collecting the finished acetum in a jar.
9) Store in labeled amber glass bottles, well-stoppered, in a cool room and out of the sunlight.

Shelf-life of dry herb aceta: The expected shelf-life for an acetum of dry herb is about 6 months. The shelf-life may be extended by the addition of 22% by volume of grain alcohol, but this would defeat the purpose if your main reason for making a pure herb acetum were to avoid the use of alcohol.

Dosage of dry herb aceta: As previously mentioned, ACV alone is not a very efficient solvent for the medicinal properties of herbs. Combined with the fact that it takes a large quantity of vinegar to cover the dried herb due to the "swelling factor," it is no surprise that these extracts are not very concentrated. The basic effective dosage is 1 tablespoonful (5 ml) taken up to 5 times daily, either straight or diluted in water. Adding a small amount of honey will assist in palatability. This is an acceptable practice for most herbs, with the exception of those taken for their bitter qualities (e.g. blue vervain, centaury, gentian, wormwood, etc.).

Basic Formula for Dry Herb Acetous Tinctures
1:5 (50A:50ACV)

Example: Celandine dry herb acetous tincture

Formula: 1:5 (50A:50ACV)
Herb weight: 100 g
Menstruum: 500 ml (composed of 250 ml grain alcohol + 250 ml apple cider vinegar)
Yield: 450 ml (measured yield after pressing and filtering)
% Return: 90%

General procedure for making dry herb acetous tinctures:

Make the menstruum by measuring and mixing the grain alcohol and the ACV in a jar, then pour it over the dry herb. Because of the alcohol content, the herb will not swell as much as it does with a dry herb acetum, and thus the acetous tincture can be made at a higher concentration (1:5 instead of 1:7). The remainder of the procedure is the same as is found under "Basic Formula for a Dry Herb Acetum." The expected shelf-life of an acetous tincture is the same as with a regular alcoholic tincture, that is, an average of about 3 years.

The primary reason for using vinegar in the menstruum is to assist in the extraction of alkaloidal constituents. In "Part 2, A Gardener's Herbal Formulary," you will find that the alkaloidal herbs celandine and ma-huang are recommended to be extracted in this manner (see the formulary for dosage recommendations). Other alkaloidal herbs, such as goldenseal and motherwort, contain different alkaloids that are readily water- and alcohol-soluble. In extracting these herbs, the addition of an acid to the menstruum becomes superfluous and is not recommended.

Basic Formula For Low-Dose, Dry Herb Acetous Tinctures
1:10 (50A:50ACV)

Certain very active herbs containing alkaloids are also best extracted with an acetous menstruum, but the formula is made intentionally weak to help prohibit overdose of the final product. The low-dose botanicals which are best extracted using a combination of alcohol and apple cider vinegar include bloodroot and lobelia.

Example: Lobelia seed acetous tincture

Formula: 1:10 (50A:50ACV)
Seed weight: 28 g (1 ounce)
Menstruum: 280 ml (composed of 140 ml grain alcohol + 140 ml apple cider vinegar)
Yield: 260 ml (measured yield after decanting and filtering)
% Return: 93%

Procedure for making lobelia seed acetous tincture:

1) Bruise the lobelia seed by grinding briefly in an electric coffee grinder or blender, or by rubbing vigorously in a mortar and pestle.
2) Put the bruised seed in a macerating container.
3) Measure and mix the grain alcohol and the ACV, then pour this menstruum over the seed.
4) Tightly cap the jar and shake the contents, label appropriately, then place on a dark shelf at room temperature, shaking daily for at least 2 weeks.
5) At the end of this time, simply allow the macerating extract to settle overnight and then decant the clear liquid slowly through a cheesecloth or coffee filter into a clean jar, leaving the slurry of seed at the bottom of the macerating jar. Note that because of the large amount of menstruum, and the fact that lobelia seed does not absorb much liquid, the extract does not require any pressing.
6) Pour the finished tincture into an amber glass jar and store in a dark and cool location. The expected shelf-life of an acetous tincture is at least 3 years.

Dosage of low-dose botanicals: The best rule of thumb for an initial adult dosage of any low-dose botanical is 5 drops of the extract, diluted in at least a cup of water. The extract may be taken 3 to 5 times per day, preferably upon waking, between meals, and just before bed. Low-dose botanicals are often mixed with other herbs in order to improve the overall effect. For instance, lobelia extract, an antispasmodic and expectorant, may be mixed with mullein extract, an emollient herb with positive effects on the mucous membranes. Low-dose botanicals usually comprise only 10% of any given formula. For example, 10 ml of lobelia acetous tincture could be combined with 90 ml of mullein tincture. The dosage of this compound is 1 to 2 droppersful (30 to 60 drops) 3 to 5 times a day or as needed to allay coughing.

Chapter 7
Herbal Glycerites

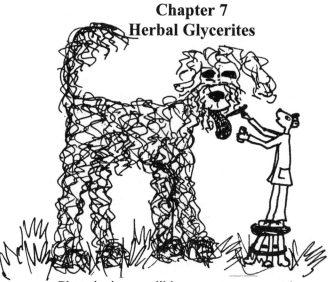

Glycerin is an edible, sweet, syrupy substance that is chemically related to alcohol.[7] It is a passable solvent and preservative and is therefore sometimes used to make alcohol-free herbal extracts. Glycerin is actually a by-product of soap and candle manufacture, where fats and oils are broken down into fatty acids and glycerin by the use of high pressure steam. Kosher grade vegetable glycerin produced from coconut oil is widely available in pharmacies and is preferred over animal-based glycerin.

Alcohol-free herbal extracts using glycerin as the primary solvent are known as glycerites. The main advantage of using glycerin instead of alcohol in extraction is to avoid the use of the alcohol. The main disadvantage is that glycerin is inferior to alcohol both as a solvent and as a preservative. Glycerites are almost always less potent than alcohol-based extracts, and they have a shorter expected shelf-life. Fresh herb glycerites are almost always superior to dry herb glycerites, since the glycerin is effective in preserving the expressed plant juices, but not particularly efficient in actually drawing constituents out of dry cell

---

[7] The molecular formula for glycerin is $C_3H_8O_3$, while the molecular formula for alcohol is C_2H_5OH.

structure. The cardinal rule in the production of glycerites is that the absolute glycerin content in the finished extract must exceed 55%. Glycerites containing less than 55% glycerin will very likely grow bacteria and go bad in storage. Like grain alcohol, vegetable glycerin is only 95% pure. When figuring the glycerin content of the finished extract, you must take into account the 5% of water contributed by the glycerin, in addition to any water added to the menstruum, and the water contributed by the plant itself. The formulas for glycerites given in this chapter and in the formulary section of this book have all been designed to ensure that the finished glycerite contains more than 55% glycerin content. Any glycerite may be rendered stable by the addition of sufficient grain alcohol to preserve it (22% of the total volume), but this would undermine the intent of purists who prefer an alcohol-free product.

You may have already divined that I am actually not much prejudiced against alcohol. The amount of alcohol consumed in the recommended daily dosage of a tincture containing alcohol is readily metabolized by a normal liver. In most cases, I use tinctures made with alcohol instead of glycerites, even when working with small children. However, extracts made with alcohol may be contraindicated for treating individuals with pre-existing liver disease, for reformed alcoholics, or for individuals who are overtly allergic to alcohol. In these cases, it is important to remember the option of using herbal teas. However, if making tea is for some reason inconvenient, using a glycerite may be a viable option. Glycerites are also widely used in veterinary practice.

Glycerin is a good solvent for tannins, and when mixed with alcohol and water in a menstruum for extracting herbs that are high in tannic acid, it will help stabilize the tincture and hold the tannins in solution. You will observe that some of the recipes in the formulary section of this book (e.g. hawthorn, meadowsweet, red root, rhubarb, self-heal, witch hazel, yellow dock, and yerba mansa) call for the addition of a small amount of glycerin to the menstruum, along with alcohol and water. Adding 10% of vegetable glycerin to the menstruum used in extracting these herbs helps prohibit precipitation of extractives and ultimately extends the shelf-life of the tincture.

Basic Formula for Fresh Herb Glycerites
1:2 (100Gly)

Example: Glycerite of fresh German chamomile flowers

Formula: 1:2 (100Gly)
Fresh herb weight: 200 g
Menstruum: 400 ml glycerin
Plant water content: 79%
Yield: 480 ml (measured yield after pressing and filtering)
% return: 86%
Absolute glycerin content of finished glycerite: 68%[8]
Convenienty, the absolute glycerin content of a finished extract
is figured in the same way as the absolute alcohol content.

To figure the absolute glycerin content of the menstruum,
multiply the volume of glycerin x .95 (absolute glycerin content of
vegetable glycerin).

400 x .95 = 380 [380 ml absolute glycerin in menstruum]

By running a drying sample, it was determined that the plant
water content of the fresh chamomile flowers was 79%. The calculated water content of the entire quantity of fresh flowers used
in the glycerite was:

200 x .79 = 158 [158 ml plant water in the batch]

To determine the total liquid available, add the volume of the
menstruum to the volume of the plant water.

400 + 158 = 558 [558 ml total liquid in the extract]

---

[8]The finished glycerin content of this extract is well above the requisite 55% glycerin content required to preserve it. This provides some
assurance that the extract will not go bad. Another significant factor
contributing to the stability of any herbal glycerite is the cleanliness of
the herbs. Inclusion of any nonherb particulate matter such as soil
should be carefully avoided since glycerin, unlike alcohol, does not
necessarily kill bacteria.

Formula to figure the absolute glycerin content (i.e. the content of pure glycerin) of the finished glycerite.

M = absolute glycerin content of the menstruum
L = total liquid
G = absolute glycerin content of the finished glycerite

$$\frac{M}{L} \times 100 = G$$

$$\frac{380}{558} \times 100 = 68$$ [68% abslolute glycerin content in the the finished extract]

* * * * * * *

Chamomile is used in this example, because fresh chamomile flowers lend themselves particularly well to extraction in glycerin. In my experience, other herbs that make exceptional glycerites include: fresh American ginseng root, dried bilberries, fresh dandelion whole plant, dried elderberries, fresh green fennel seeds, fresh mint leaves, fresh mullein flowers, fresh stevia leaves, fresh echinacea roots, and fresh valerian roots. The formulas for these glycerites are all listed in "Part 2, A Gardener's Herbal Formulary."

General procedure for making fresh herb glycerites:

1) Weigh the fresh herb and put it in a blender.
2) Measure the glycerin.
3) Pour the glycerin over the herb and blend thoroughly.
4) Pour the slurry into a macerating container.
5) Cover tightly, shake, and set to macerate in a dark place at room temperature. Label with date and herb name.
6) Shake daily for a period of 2 weeks. At the end of this time, pour the macerating glycerite into a pressing cloth and express thoroughly, either by hand or with a tincture press.
7) Collect the crude glycerite in a jar, label, and set it on a shelf to settle for 2 or more days. Extended settling time is recommended due to the high viscosity of glycerites.
8) After the solids have settled to the bottom of the jar, decant the clear liquid through several layers of clean cheesecloth and collect the finished glycerite in a jar.
9) Store the glycerite in labeled amber glass bottles, well-stoppered, in a cool room, out of the sunlight. Fresh herb glycerites have an expected shelf-life of at least 1 year.

Dosage of glycerites: Considering that glycerin is substantially less efficient than alcohol as a solvent, it makes sense to double the tincture dosage when administering glycerites. In other words, if the starting dosage for an alcoholic extract were 30 drops 5 times a day, you would probably have to use 60 drops of the glycerite 5 times a day to get the same effect.

Comparing alcoholic tinctures to glycerites: Herbalists are able to compare the relative strength of glycerine- vs. alcohol-based extracts when they use them in phytotherapy. Your child is coming down with a cold, you give her echinacea glycerite, she goes out to play and . . . somehow the cold never shows up! Analytical studies can also demonstrate the relative efficiency of extraction provided by glycerites vs. tinctures. A liquid chromatograph coupled to a mass spectrometer can be quite useful. Studies of this sort show, for instance, that the various isoquinoline alkaloids in Goldenseal (*Hydrastis canadensis*) are extracted about half as well by a glycerine-water mixture as with alcohol and water.

Chapter 8
Teas and Decoctions

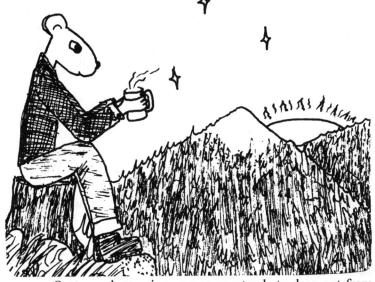

On towards evening, my energy tends to drop out from under me, and if some vagrant bacterium or virus is trying to take hold, this is when I begin to notice it. Of course, herbalists do not get sick, they simply exercise their immune systems, but on this particular night my immunity definitely was being challenged. I kept shuffling around the seed house, closing up, gathering cups, turning out lights, and locking the doors of side-rooms, allowing myself a dejected sniff or two. When I walked into the commons area, grateful for the heat still radiating from the benevolent black wood stove, the top of my head was swept by one of the bundles of thyme hanging from a beam in the roof. These bundles had been there since late fall, when we finally had dug out a few of the old gentlemen plants, which had so resolutely lined the drive-way for a decade. The plants were composed more of dead wood than live, but it was a little sad to dig them up—not only because they had served us (and the bees) so well, but because a few of the bottom branches were still lively and trying to survive by rooting in the rocky soil. Feeling like heartless cads, we dug them out to make room for new plants, put the old wood and roots in the compost pile, and tied the live branches together to hang in the seed house. There they stayed, longer than necessary, nearly dry to start with and now as dry as mummies. I wondered if the herb still would be good, but then flashed on the old tradition, hatched before the invention of cellophane bags, of keeping herbs in the rafters of the hut until they were needed.

So, distracted for a moment from self-pity and stimulated by my native herbal curiosity, I took down a bundle and gave it an experimental shake. It let go of a plume of house dust that had accumulated on the slightly sticky leaves, but it also gave off its characteristically wholesome fragrance. Now fully sidetracked from closing up, I cleared a place on the table, set out a sturdy screen, and began rolling the bundles of thyme back and forth on the screen. I set the naked stems aside to use as fire-starter and let the dark green leaf pile up on the table beneath my screen, pushing it to the side when I needed more room. Having finished with the last bundle, I thought it would be a good idea to try to get some of the undesirable dust out of the herb, so I carefully pushed the pile off the edge of the table into a smaller-holed screen and gave it a shake over the floor. This process sacrificed a little herbal dust, but the house dust also came filtering out. I shook until the herb would give no more. Then I poured the leaves into a cellophane bag, secured it with a twist, and finished closing up the building, eventually leaving by the side door and making my way to the house with the bulging bag of thyme tucked in the crook of my arm.

The cats, who had spent the day leisurely soaking up the thin sunshine, now crouched on the low roof, wailing like starving waifs. Thoroughly self-absorbed and caring not a bit for how I was feeling, they would need to be fed immediately. I scooped dry cat food out of the bag, setting some out in bowls on the benches in the old greenhouse and tossing the remainder up on the roof where certain cats, including always the part-Siamese named Mozart, insisted on eating. It was cold inside the house. I threw some cedar kindling and a few lengths of madrone into the wood stove. The rest of the family would be coming home soon, so I put on a pot of brown rice and filled a kettle of water for making tea. Beginning to wash a few dishes, I was quick to give up when the teapot began to sing. This was my opportunity to nurture myself, and I was going to take full advantage of it. Situating a clean quart canning jar on the counter, I put a scant handful of the thyme herb into it. When the boiling water splashed over the herb, the color turned an immediate and promising green. I lidded the steaming jar with a saucer and waited, my hands on the edge of the counter, watching the currents of hot water interact with the leaves of the herb. Making tea, I mused, is a process wherein a dry and quiescent herb is converted, in a flicker of time, into a lively and congenial beverage. Transformations of this kind contain an element of magic, the magic that arises when form changes, suspending perhaps our concepts of solid reality, inviting faith, making the way for healing . . .

The wood stove crackled and popped as I sat cross-legged before it, there in the darkened living room. The tea was good, and I sipped it hot. Whether it was the rest, the satisfaction of hearing Mozart crunching kibbles on the roof, or the influence of the herbs coursing through my system I will never know, but I started feeling better and gave a sigh of relief, exhaling odors of thyme. After another moment, I got up to check on the rice. Come to think of it, I never did get sick.

Tea

Simple tea is a water extract of herbs, sometimes known as an "infusion." A good method is to pour hot water over a tablespoonful (1 to 2 g) of ground or chopped dried herbs in a cup, cover and allow to steep for 5 to 10 minutes, then strain and sip at leisure. Various "standard formulas" have been proposed for making a pot of tea; these are generally expressed as a weight:volume ratio (W:V).[9] A few of the popular ratios are: 1:16 (1 oz. dried herb:16 ozs. of water); 1:32 (1 oz. dried herb: 32 ozs. of water); and a metric formula that matches neither of these, 1:20 (50 g dried herb:1000 ml water).

---

[9]In our antiquated avoirdupois system, this W:V ratio is expressed as ozs. dry weight:ozs. fluid volume, which works out fairly well since 1 oz. dry weight (28.4 g) is reasonably equivalent to 1 oz. fluid volume (29.6 ml). Metric W:V ratios are more accurate, given that 1 ml of water weighs exactly 1 g.

Given the variation in standard formulas, the variation in the quality and particle size of herbal ingredients, and the bare fact that almost no one bothers to weigh and measure their tea ingredients anyway, the quantity of herb and water used to make the tea is best regulated with an eye toward making a palatable preparation, which is nonetheless strong enough to do the desired work. Of course, not all medicinal herbs taste good; many are bitter, some soapy, and some taste, as my wife once commented, "like dirt and twigs."

Tea Made with Fresh Herbs

There is something particularly pleasing and delightful about making tea with fresh leaves and flowers. A simple procedure is to finely mince the freshly harvested herbs, place in a quart jar, add just-boiled water, put on a lid, and let the tea stand until it is cool enough to drink. The tea can be strained into cups or sipped "right off the top." In order to create a strong effect, you will have to pack the fresh herbs into the jar, because extraction is not as efficient as with dry herbs, where the cell structure has become brittle and vulnerable to extraction through dehydration. A few herbs that extract well in the fresh form are angelica, calendula, catnip, clover, dandelion, gentian, horehound, lemon balm, lovage, self-heal, and thyme. The colors of the leaves and flowers in the jar, as well as the colors imparted to the liquid itself, are vibrant in a manner unattainable with dried herbs.

Cold Infusions

Some herbs, such as marshmallow and blessed thistle, lend their active principles better to cold water than to hot. This is usually due to the presence of mucilage or bitter principles that are denatured, to a certain extent, by boiling water. Although the quantities of herb used in making a cold infusion may be dictated by taste, the basic formula is 1:32 (W:V) (i.e. 1 oz. dried herb: 32 ozs. of water). The dried herb is slightly moistened, tied loosely in cheesecloth, and suspended just beneath the surface of cold water in a jar. The string may be draped over the edge and secured by loosely screwing on the cap, in order to keep the "tea bag" near the surface of the water. Efficient cold extraction depends on the principle of circulatory displacement.

Fresh, clear water flows through the tea bag, becomes suffused with heavy extractives and circulates downward, displacing clear water that is, in turn, forced up toward the waiting herb. In this manner, a salutary tea is created overnight.

Decoctions

A decoction is basically a simmered tea—a method of preparation best employed for the extraction of hard roots, barks, and seeds. These do not readily give up their constituents to a simple infusion. Decoctions may be taken internally, or used in baths or as an external wash. My preferred method of preparation is to put a good handful (~30 g) of the dried herbs in a quart of cold water in a saucepan, cover, and set aside for at least an hour (or even overnight) allowing the herbs to soak up as much water as possible. Then, I slowly bring the water to a low boil and simmer the herbs for 15 minutes. After straining, the decoction may be used hot or allowed to cool before use.

For those who prefer a more exact measure, a basic decoction may be made at a concentration of 1:32 (W:V) (i.e. 1 oz. dried herb:32 ozs. of water). The approximate metric equivalent is 30 g of dried herb to 1 L of water. Regardless of how you measure it, the procedure is the same as above, except that when a standard concentration is desired, the decoction is measured directly after straining, and sufficient hot water is poured back through the herb in the strainer to bring the volume back up to 1 quart (or 1 L). This replaces the water volume lost through evaporation and absorption during the process and washes any remaining goodness out of the marc.

Strong decoctions: A strong decoction may be produced by doubling the amount of herbs used, and keeping the water quantity constant (i.e. 60 g of dried herb to 1 L of water). Another method of producing a strong decoction is to make a basic decoction (30 g of dried herb to 1 L of water), strain into a clean saucepan, and simmer very slowly until the volume is reduced by half (to 500 ml). As the decoction thickens, the liquid must be stirred frequently in order to prevent burning. Strong decoctions are of use in making compresses and soaks and in making herbal syrups (see "Chapter 11, Poultices, Compresses, and Soaks" and "Chapter 9, Herbal Succi and Syrups").

Finally, if the decoction is simmered slowly and stirred constantly, the water may be evaporated off altogether, leaving a concentrated, gummy substance known as a "soft extract." This method has been commonly employed for making throat lozenges using horehound or licorice.

Dosage of teas and decoctions: As with other forms of herb intake, the size, strength, and frequency of dosage of strong medicinal herbs in tea form is best regulated according to the body weight and sensitivity of the individual and according to the severity of the illness. The normal effective dosage is 2 or 3 cups of an infusion or decoction per day. It is interesting to note that according to the physiomedical tradition,[10] in the treatment of acute conditions where a high dosage was required, an infusion or decoction was considered to be the best treatment by far. Indeed, in most cases a normal dose of tincture contains far fewer extractives than does a cup of strong tea, even considering the superiority of alcohol as a solvent. In the case of pernicious infection, the teas need to be made strong and the patient cajoled into drinking as much as possible, and as often as possible. For treating less acute conditions such as mild adrenal imbalance, the tea generally would be made much weaker and taken only once or twice daily over a period of several weeks in order to help correct the condition.

The water extract of certain very pungent and stimulating herbs such as cayenne pepper or yerba mansa may be made very dilute, taken a half cup at a time and still provide ample effect. Low-dose botanicals such as blue flag, lobelia, and wild indigo certainly must be approached with great caution in regard to the

---

[10]Physiomedical tradition: A system of herbal medicine developed in the mid to late 19th century based on the belief that each individual carries an inherent "vital force," a kind of cellular intelligence capable of orchestrating physiological functions. Disease symptoms were considered to be an expression of the body attempting to rid itself of toxins, and herbs were administered to help stimulate elimination of toxins, tonify the organs, and restore the system to equilibrium.

quantity of herb used in making the tea or decoction and the eventual dosage. Failure to recognize the highly active effects of these herbs can lead to overstimulation of the physiological response, resulting sometimes in allergic reaction or vomiting.

Other low-dose botanicals such as arnica, bloodroot, celandine, or juniper berries contain potentially acrid substances. Overdose of these can lead to irritation of the mucous membranes. For these reasons, it is preferable to use low-dose botanicals in the form of a tincture, which can be accurately measured by the drop and administered by diluting in at least a cup of water.

Storing teas and decoctions: Water extracts of herbs are not preserved in any way and must be made anew each day. Simple infusions are best made up as needed, by the cupful or by the pot. Cold infusions can be made using a pint jar if a very small quantity is desired. The recipe for a decoction can also be cut in half to produce only a pint of finished extract, which may be utilized in a single day without waste.

Milk as an additive to tea: Milk, whether produced from organic cows or goats, is a nutritive and demulcent substance. It combines well with many kinds of tea and can improve palatability (e.g. German chamomile tea with milk). In this case, the bitter digestive and sedative properties of the tea are not compromised, but rather augmented by the addition of milk, and the taste is improved. However, the addition of milk is not always indicated. Of course, lactose-intolerant individuals will want to avoid dairy. And, when treating upper respiratory infection, the use of clear teas is advised. Milk only serves to increase the production of mucous, which harbors bacteria. Excessive mucous causes discomfort and congestion. It would not make sense to add milk to an infusion of thyme leaf meant as a treatment for sore throat, congestion, and cough.

The proteins in milk bind with tannins and render them inactive. Tannins are very significant medicinal agents, demonstrating antioxidant, antiseptic, and astringent properties. For example, green tea, self-heal, and witch hazel all owe their medicinal effects to tannins. Therefore, in making a decoction of witch hazel to be used as a gargle for treating sore throat, one

71

would not add milk, because milk nullifies the desired astringency of the decoction.

However, tannins are not always beneficial. If taken in excess, they can be constipating, and they can cause stomach upset. In this case, adding milk will help neutralize excessive tannins in medicinal teas. For example, the addition of milk to black tea makes it kinder to the stomach, without compromising the stimulating effects of the alkaloid caffeine.

Sweeteners: Adding sugar or honey to tea can improve palatability, but it can also subvert the activity of herbs. For example, wormwood, employed for its bitter digestive and antiparasitic effects, is best taken as a straight, unadulterated infusion. In fact, given the predominance of bland, fatty, salty, and sweet foods in the typical modern diet, it makes sense to use bitter and sour herbs in their naked and natural state. Avoiding sugar in the diet is especially significant for those suffering blood sugar imbalance, cancer, candidiasis, excessive stomach acid, or infections.

* * * * * * *

Making tea is steeped in tradition and this simple liquid is probably the progenitor of all types of medicinal preparations. I can imagine the original mother of the wise woman tradition, on her knees grinding fresh leaves in a stone mortar. She adds a little water, stirs it around with her finger, cups some in her hand, takes a sip, makes a face, then squats back on her haunches and mutters the cave-equivalent of "pretty good!" Tea is made of water, the same life-giving substance of which people are made. Water alone washes the system of toxins. The act of stopping your busy life, preparing the infusion, sitting, drinking, and even perhaps daydreaming with cup in hand, are all part of the healing.

Chapter 9
Herbal Succi and Syrups

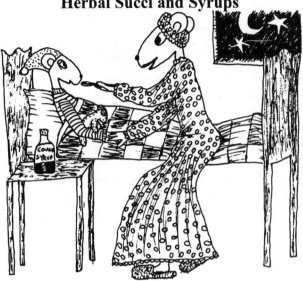

An herbal succus (Latin for "juice;" the plural is succi) is simply plant juice, best obtained by grinding, blending, or mashing the fresh plant and then slowly expressing the juice under high pressure in a good tincture press. The juice is then preserved by the addition of a little alcohol—just enough to make the finished absolute alcohol content measure above 20%, which is requisite for preservation purposes. The best herbs for making succi are those that traditionally have been used in the fresh state, are of high water content, and relinquish their juices freely under pressure. Herbs chosen for making a succus must contain water-soluble active principles, since the alcohol is not available for extraction, but is employed solely for preservation. The primary reason for making an herbal extract in this way is to maximize the volume of actual plant juice in the extract while minimizing the alcohol content. The following are good examples of fresh herbs that can be used to make succi: calendula, chickweed, cleavers, dandelion, gotu kola, jewelweed, jiao-gu-lan, lemon balm, nettles, plantain, purslane, skullcap, and violet. These herbs are typified by the presence of water-soluble constituents and succulent tissues. As long as you keep these requirements in mind, you may choose other herbs for making effective succi.

Basic Formula for Fresh Herb Succi

3:1

(3 parts herbal juice by volume:1 part grain alcohol by volume)

Example: Fresh dandelion root succus

500 g of fresh dandelion roots are mashed and pressed to yield 315 ml of juice.

Adding the alcohol: 315 divided by 3 = 105

105 ml of grain alcohol is now added to the juice in order to preserve it. The extract is agitated in order to mix the alcohol and the juice.

Total available liquid: 315 ml juice + 105 ml alcohol = 420 ml

Settling and filtering: Set the succus aside for 3 days to settle. After settling, decant through cheesecloth or a paper filter.

Yield: 350 ml.

% Return: 83%

Note that approximately 17% of the total available liquid was lost during the filtering process.

Final absolute alcohol content of the succus: 24%

To determine the final absolute alcohol content multiply the volume of grain alcohol (105 ml) x 0.95 (absolute alcohol content of grain alcohol) = 99.75 ml (volume of absolute alcohol available to this extract). 99.75 divided by 420 (total available liquid) = 0.238, which is rounded to 24%.

Basic procedure for making fresh herb succi:

1) Grind the fresh herb in a suitable mill, food processor, juicer, blender, or mortar and pestle until it is reduced to a mash. Make sure to collect any juice that flows freely from the herb during this process.

2) Immediately slop the mashed herb into a pressing cloth and begin pressing in a tincture press. Express the juice slowly, starting at very low pressure and gradually increasing the pressure. Mucilaginous herbs (e.g. dandelion and purslane) must be pressed very slowly, while herbs with thin and freely-flowing juice (e.g. gotu kola and lemon balm) will press out more quickly.

3) Collect the expressed juice in a wide-mouthed jar.

4) When the mashed herb ceases yielding liquid, measure the volume of the juice and divide by 3. Slowly pour this quantity of grain alcohol into the juice and agitate.

5) Allow the succus to settle in a lidded jar for several days, then decant the clear juice through a paper filter or at least 4 layers of cheesecloth. Succi are infamous for producing copious quantities of sludge, which is the reason for the long settling time and the slowness of filtration.

6) Keep the filtered succus in correctly labeled, amber bottles, tightly stoppered and stored out of the light. The expected shelf-life of herbal succi is approximately 2 years.

Dosage of herbal succi: Due to the low alcohol content and consequent lack of "sting," herbal succi are commonly used as a direct and undiluted external application to mucous membranes or to oily skin, acne, wounds, contusions, sutures or incisions. To reduce further the chance of stinging, the extract may be diluted in water at the rate of 2 droppersful (60 drops) in 1 cup (240 ml) of water and applied immediately as a wash to the injured parts. Used internally, the adult dosage of succi is the same as for tinctures: 1 to 2 droppersful (30 to 60 drops) diluted in a little water and taken 3 to 5 times daily, depending on the urgency of the problem being addressed. It may be of benefit to increase the amount and/or frequency of intake of certain gentle and harmless herbs, such as chickweed, dandelion, gotu kola, or lemon balm, in order to amplify the effect.

Herbal Syrups

Traditionally, herbal syrups are made by combining 2 parts of sugar by weight with 1 part of water extract (strong tea or decoction) by volume. For example, 500 grams of sugar are combined with 250 ml of a concentrated tea or decoction, dissolved over gentle heat, while stirring constantly, until the sugar dissolves, in order to produce medicated syrup. This syrup carries the active constituents of the herb in a very agreeable form that generally meets with enthusiastic patient compliance. The product is fully preserved, but subject to crystallization. I personally prefer herbal syrups made with raw honey instead of sugar.

Honey (Latin: *Mel*)

Honey makes a very good carrier for cough medicines and for laxatives. It is also an acceptable carrier for many other herbs with the exception of bitter herbs, since, in this case, the effects are dependent largely upon the bitter taste.

Honey is the nectar of flowers, transformed by the honeybee *(Apis mellifera)* into a sweet secretion that is deposited into the honey-comb of the hive. Honey is, in and of itself, a syrup composed of fructose, glucose, water, proteins (such as pollen), enzymes, minerals, and the ethereal essence of flowers. The acidity of honey lies between pH3 and pH6—a relatively acidic substance.

Raw honey is herein defined as honey extracted from the honeycomb by means of centrifuge or gentle heat not to exceed 110° F. Heated above this temperature, honey is quickly divested of its innate medicinal virtues and fragrance. Raw honey is subject to crystallization in storage. If this occurs, it may be reliquified by setting the jar in a pan of hot water not to exceed 110° F.

Medicinal virtues of raw honey: Used externally, honey may be applied to the face as an antimicrobial and healing treatment for acne or other skin eruptions. Simply rub into the face just prior to showering. The complexion becomes clear, and the skin is moistened and softened, attaining a healthy sheen. Honey is also an excellent topical treatment for burns and supperative infections—even gangrene. Sterile gauze bandages are soaked in honey and layered on the affected area. The bandages are renewed several times daily. The influence is antibiotic, and healing is accelerated. This therapy also results in reduced formation of scar tissue.

Honey alone is a traditional treatment for upset stomach, heartburn, and the gastritis caused by overindulgence in alcoholic beverages. The influence is calmative, warming, moistening, and healing. Honey also inhibits the growth of *Helicobacter pylori,* the organism that plays a role in the formation of gastric ulcers.

Honey contains pollen grains from a wide array of local plants. Daily use of locally manufactured honey results in improved immunity to local allergens, such as airborne pollen from trees, grasses, and flowers. The mode of activity is homeopathic—

small quantities of the allergen cue the individual to produce the appropriate antibodies. Many people find relief from allergy symptoms (such as runny nose, itchy eyes, and sneezing) by simply adding raw local honey to their morning tea. In every case, the beneficial activity of raw honey may be augmented by combining it with herbs, and one of the best ways to accomplish this is by means of herbal syrups made with honey.

Formula for Basic Herbal Syrups made with Honey
1:2

(1 part water extract of herbs by volume:2 parts honey by volume)

General procedure for making herbal syrups:

1) Make a strong tea or decoction of the desired herb(s).
2) Strain, measure the liquid, and pour into a saucepan or double-boiler.
3) Add 2 times the volume of pure honey. Stirring continuously, heat the mixture until it incorporates completely. The temperature of the honey should not exceed 110° F. Do not simmer or boil. High temperatures will denature the honey.
4) Remove the hot syrup from the heat and pour into sterilized canning jars.
5) Cap tightly with sterilized lids, label appropriately, and store in a cool, dry place, out of the light.
6) Syrup made in this manner has an expected shelf-life of 1 year. Keep opened containers under refrigeration. The syrup must be discarded if mold appears on the surface.

Example 1: Syrup of violet leaf and flower

Make a strong decoction of dried violet leaves and flowers by soaking 60 g of the herb overnight in 1 L of cold water and, in the morning, simmering for 15 minutes, then straining to produce 800 ml of strong decoction. Combine the decoction with 1600 ml of honey, heat gently, and stir until the liquids incorporate perfectly, then pour off into sterilized jars.

Violet syrup is a strong alterative, a specific treatment for oral cancers. Violet syrup is also a useful treatment for the cough of children and toddlers over the age of 12 months.

Example 2: Compound cough syrup of spikenard
Procedure and formula

1) Make a strong decoction of spikenard by adding 60 g of sliced, dried roots to 1000 ml of water, soaking overnight, and in the morning, bringing the water to a low boil and simmering for 15 minutes. After straining, the decoction is measured to 800 ml.
2) In a saucepan or double boiler, combine the 800 ml of spikenard decoction with 1,600 ml of honey and heat over a low fire, stirring constantly until the ingredients are thoroughly incorporated. Do not simmer or boil.
3) The volume is now 2,400 ml. Pour the syrup into sterilized jars, leaving a little room for adding the tinctures.
4) Tinctures are now added in order to augment the effects of this preparation. A compound tincture is made by combining lobelia acetous extract and elecampane tincture at the rate of 1:9 (1 part lobelia:9 parts elecampane). Add 1 part by volume (120 ml) of this compound tincture to 20 parts by volume (2,400 ml) of spikenard syrup.
5) After adding the compound tincture in equally divided portions to all the jars of syrup, the jars are capped and shaken in order to mix in the tincture.
6) Label appropriately and store in a cool, dry place, out of the light.

This strong preparation of spikenard (*Aralia californica* or *A. racemosa*), elecampane, and lobelia is useful for fighting upper respiratory infection, arresting cough, and strengthening the upper respiratory tract. The basic adult dosage is 1 tablespoon as needed, up to 5 times per day.

Syrup Made from Reduced Berries
Elderberry syrup procedure and formula

1) Use 1 cup of dried black elderberries (weighs ~100 g)
2) Place the dried berries in a bowl and add 2 cups of boiling water. Cover with a plate and allow to sit overnight.
3) In the morning, pour the softened berries into a blender and vortex them into a mush.

4) Pour the berry mixture into a fine sieve and press it through with your fingers, or press it out in a tincture press. Either of these methods will separate the juice from the seeds. Save the juice, and compost the seeds.

5) The volume of the juice is now 2 cups. Simmer the juice on the back of the stove at low heat, stirring frequently. Keep reducing the juice until it reaches half volume (1 cup). This takes 1 to 2 hours. The juice is now very concentrated with pectin and bioactive compounds.

6) Stir in 1 cup raw honey or glycerine, bringing the total volume back up to 2 cups. This is a thick syrup!

7) Filter through 4 layers of cheesecloth. Squeeze out the cheesecloth by hand, thereby recovering all the juice but excluding errant skins, seeds, and undesirable solids.

8) Bottle the syrup in amber tincture bottles or jars. The glycerin preparation may be stored in a cool place out of the light, while the honey preparation is probably best kept refrigerated. The shelf-life is 1 year.

Elderberry syrup may also be made from fresh black elderberries. Place the berries in a saucepan with a little water and set to the back of the stove on low heat. Stirring frequently, cook until the berries are throughly softened, then remove from heat and allow to cool until they can be comfortably handled. Press out in a tincture press or pass through a large sieve, thereby excluding the seeds. Collect the juice and compost the seeds. Return the juice to the saucepan and set to the back of the stove on low heat, stirring frequently. Reduce to ¼ the original volume, producing a thick juice (this may take all day). Measure, and add an equal volume of vegetable glycerine or honey. Filter and bottle as above.

Over the years, I have learned to rely heavily on the syrup of black elderberries as a preventative and treatment for the common cold and influenza. I've noticed that many children balk at taking bitter medicines, but freely accept elderberry syrup, and are really helped by it, as it gives them some protection from the inevitable virus that lurks around the schoolyard like a bad kid bent on mischief. This syrup is so tasty that it is best stored beyond the reach of those who would take it too freely!

Honeyed roots: Most raw, soft-fleshed roots can be made into a delicious sweet by simmering them in honey. Although this process denatures the honey, it increases the warming and moistening power of the herbs. Wash the roots, peel if necessary, then thinly slice. Place a single layer of slices in a small saucepan and add 3 tablespoons of honey. Bring the honey to a simmer on a low flame, and keep it there for a few minutes. The honey will froth up around the roots and keep frothing. Remove from the heat and allow to cool slightly. Return to heat and bring back to a simmer. Repeat several times, until the roots are cooked and suffused with honey. Honeyed roots may be made up as needed, with medicinality in accordance with the attributes of the herb being used. In this manner, we have made excellent sweets of burdock, elecampane, ginseng, horseradish, marshmallow (yum!), dang-shen, and yellow dock.

Sunny honey: Certain aromatic herbs may be made into an herbal honey simply by packing a jar or crock full of fresh flowers, then covering with honey and leaving indoors, on a sunny windowsill, allowing to macerate for 2 weeks time. Then, press the honey/herb mixture through a cheesecloth or in a pressing bag in a tincture press, and collect the herbal honey and use as-is. This can be a great way to make a cough syrup out of bergamot, fennel, horehound, hyssop, lemon balm, osha roots, tulsi, or any other herb or root that contains aromatic fixed or essential oils.

Contraindications: Raw (uncooked) honey and herbal syrups made from uncooked honey should not be given to infants aged less than 12 months. In rare cases, honey can be contaminated with spores of the bacterium *Clostridium botulinum,* which can proliferate in the immature intestine, causing infant botulism. This, in some cases, is fatal. Also, honey produced in areas where transgenic (GMO) crops are being grown should be avoided like the plague, due to the potential content of aberrant allergens.

Chapter 10
Herbal Oils, Salves, and Creams

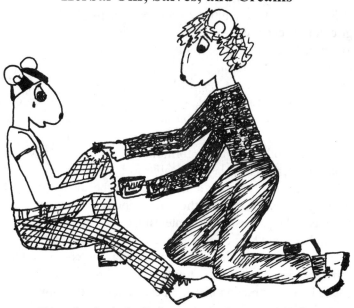

To make herbal oil (sometimes known as infused oil), fresh or dried herbs are steeped for a period of time in vegetable oil using gentle heat to assist the extraction. This process is sometimes known as "digestion," because the slow process of deriving the medicinal agents from the herbs is likened to the physiological process of deriving nutrients from foods. Over time, warm oil efficiently extracts certain medicinal compounds from herbs. Gums, resins, and oleoresins are highly soluble in warm oil. Alkaloids, essential oils, mucilage, and other active principles (e.g. the hypericins of Saint John's wort) are also at least partially soluble in oil.

It must be understood that *infused herbal oils* are not *pure essential oils*. Pure essential oils are extracted from the plant with steam distillation, are diluted prior to use, and used in much smaller dosage than are infused oils.

Herbal oils are used externally, massaged directly into the skin, or sometimes dropped sparingly into the ears. Herbal oils are also the primary ingredient for making salves and creams. Oils are absorbed directly through the skin into the body.

Oil

Unfortunately, vegetable oil is not only a good extractive medium for certain soluble constituents of plants, but also for agricultural chemicals—including pesticides and herbicides. Cottonseed oil is particularly suspect for this reason. If the oil is not organically certified, you take your chances that it may be laced with chemicals. Organically certified olive oil is probably the best choice for making herbal oils, although other cold-pressed fixed oils such as jojoba, sesame, or almond oil may also be used.

The following basic formulas for herbal oil, salve, and cream are designed to be applicable to a wide range of herbs. Although an impromptu oil infusion may be made simply by covering the herb with oil in the macerating vessel, measuring the ingredients helps ensure the integrity of the finished product. Certain herbs are best dried and crushed or ground up before oil extraction. These include arnica, calendula, and comfrey. Other herbs are best used fresh, thinly sliced, bruised, or coarsely ground before extracting in oil. These include elder, figwort, and Saint John's wort.

"Part 2, A Gardener's Herbal Formulary" gives specific information on which herbs extract well in oil, what plant parts are used, and whether the plants are best used in the fresh or the dry state. The reader is therefore referred to the formulary section in order to identify more herbs that can be processed according to these basic formulas.

Basic Formula for Fresh Herb Infused Oils
1:3
(fresh herb weight in g:oil volume in ml)

Example: Infused oil of fresh figwort leaves

100 g fresh figwort leaves
300 ml olive oil

This oil is very good for treating swollen lymph nodes, old burns, ulcerations, wounds, and abrasions. The oil may be used as-is or as an ingredient for making salve or cream.

General procedure for making infused oil of fresh herbs:

1) Finely mince the fresh herb by slicing it with a knife on a cutting board. Weigh and then place the herb in a macerating vessel (quart jar, gallon jar, or crockpot).
2) Cover with the measured oil and stir thoroughly. The herb-oil mixture must be maintained at a temperature of 110° to 120° F (43° to 49° C) for a period of 1 week (2 weeks for Saint John's wort). Stir daily.
3) When the time allotted for the infusion is over, pour off the warm herb-oil mixture through several layers of cheesecloth into a bowl, squeezing the herb in the cheesecloth to further express the oil. A tincture press may be used, but it also forces water from the plant, water which must subsequently be excluded.
4) Pour the crude oil into a clean, dry jar. Cover, and allow it to stand undisturbed overnight. Particulate matter and water will settle out to the bottom of the jar.
5) The next morning, carefully decant the oil through several layers of cheesecloth into another clean, dry jar, leaving the watery sludge behind in the bottom of the settling jar. Do this by pouring the clear oil off the top. Discard the sludge.
6) Store the finished herbal oil in tightly stoppered, correctly labeled, amber glass bottles in a cool place and out of the light. Properly made, fresh herb infused oils require the addition of no preservatives, and they have an expected shelf-life of at least 1 year.

Source of Heat

A crockpot works best for maintaining a constant, low temperature. Do not try to make herbal oils on the stove top, as higher temperatures ruin the herb and denature the oil. To use a crockpot, put the ingredients directly into the ceramic vessel and check the temperature of the digesting oil by suspending a thermometer in it, adjusting the thermostat on the crockpot to maintain the oil between 110° to 120° F (43° to 49° C). During extraction, leave the crockpot or jar lid cracked open so that plant water can evaporate.

Most crockpots have only a rudimentary thermostat (low and high), and the lowest setting is usually too hot for herbal oils. You can modify the crockpot by installing a dimmer switch on its electric cord. Have someone who understands electricity do this, with safety in mind. Dimmer switches are available at hardware stores (designed for use on lights) and, when used in conjunction with a crockpot, they allow infinite tuning of the temperature. You can experiment by filling the crockpot with water and fiddling with the knob on the dimmer switch until the proper temperature is achieved. This way, you won't sacrifice your first herbal oil on the altar of science.

The oil may also be made in a wide-mouth quart or gallon jar using other sources of heat such as the sun, a wood stove, a furnace, or an oven set at 110°. It helps to insulate the jar by placing it in a shallow pan of water. This also will serve to catch the oil if the jar accidentally breaks.

If the source of heat is sporadic (e.g. heat from the sun or a wood stove) and the oil is allowed to cool at times during the digestion process, the contents may begin to ferment. This can sour the final product. Fermentation will be visible as active bubbling of the ingredients. To arrest fermentation, heat the herb-oil mixture in a saucepan or crockpot, raising the temperature to 150° F (65° C). Stir constantly until all bubbling ceases. Then cool the mixture back down to the digesting temperature and complete the extraction in the normal manner.

Do not try processing herbal oils in a blender. This practice will create an undesirable emulsification of the plant water and oil.

Basic Formula for Dry Herb Infused Oils
1:5
(dry herb weight in g:oil volume in ml)

Example 1: Arnica oil

100 g dried and coarsely ground arnica blossoms
500 ml olive oil

This oil is sometimes known as "arnicated oil." It is an excellent penetrating anti-inflammatory for treating traumatic injuries such as bruises, sprains, and torn ligaments. Arnica resolves stuck blood.

Example 2: Calendula oil

100 g dried and coarsely ground calendula blossoms
500 ml olive oil

This oil is sometimes known as "calendulated oil." It is a good antiseptic and healing agent for treating cuts, scrapes, chapped skin, diaper rash, eczema, and windburn.

Example 3: Comfrey root oil

100 g dried and coarsely ground comfrey roots
500 ml olive oil

This oil is best used for speeding healing of broken bones, shallow wounds, scratches, diaper rash, abraded or wind-burned skin, etc.

Example 4: Goldenseal leaf oil

100 g dried and coarsely ground goldenseal leaves, picked after the berries ripen
500 ml olive oil

This oil is best used as an antibacterial for treating wounds, and is also healing to traumatized or infected mucous membranes.

General procedure for making dry herb infused oils:

1) Finely crush the dried herb by rubbing it through a screen or grind it to a coarse powder.

2) Weigh the herb and place it in the macerating vessel.

3) Measure the oil and pour it over the dried herb. Stir thoroughly, until the herb is completely incorporated into the oil.

4) Maintain the digesting oil at a temperature of 110° to 120° F (43° to 49° C) for a period of 2 weeks. The use of a crockpot is highly recommended, but other sources of heat are acceptable. Keep dry herb infusions out of the direct sunlight. Since there is no water in the herb, there is no danger of fermentation in the process. The herb will have a tendency to settle into a gummy clump at the bottom of the vessel, so extraction is improved by stirring several times per day.

5) Press the oil. Using a tincture press is highly recommended, because unlike fresh herbs that tend to repel the oil, the dry herb will have absorbed much oil during the 2-week digestion. The oil yields slowly from the herb; therefore, press at low pressure to start and gradually increase the pressure as the herb gives up the oil. Finish at high pressure.

6) Pour the crude oil into a clean, dry jar. Put on the lid and allow the oil to stand undisturbed overnight. A heavy sludge will settle out to the bottom of the jar. The next morning, carefully decant the oil through several layers of cheesecloth into another clean, dry jar, leaving the sludge behind in the bottom of the settling jar.

7) Store the finished herbal oil in a correctly labeled, tightly stoppered, amber glass bottle in a cool place and out of the light. Properly made, dry herb infused oils require the addition of no preservatives, and they have an expected shelf-life of at least 2 years.

Basic Formula for Herbal Salves
100:17
(volume of herbal oil in ml:weight of beeswax in g)

Example 1: Trauma salve

500 ml calendula oil
250 ml arnica oil
250 ml Saint John's wort oil
170 g beeswax pieces, melted

Trauma salve is useful for treating bruises, deep muscle injury, and sprains.

Note: Beeswax is a natural product that is universally applicable for making salves and creams. In herbal manufacture, beeswax is considered to be much superior to paraffin, which is derived from petroleum.

General procedure for making herbal salves:

1) Measure and combine the herbal oils by pouring them into a double boiler or a crockpot. Bring the temperature of the oil up to 150° F (65° C).
2) On a tabletop or counter, somewhat removed from the stove area, set out a sufficient number of dry, clean, and appropriately labeled salve tins, salve jars, or other shallow glass jars—in all enough to accept the volume of salve being made.
3) In a separate double boiler, slowly melt the wax until it is fluid. This can be done in a saucepan directly over a very low burner, but the pan should be hand-held and given constant attention to make sure it isn't overheating. Wax eventually will ignite if left unattended on a burner.
4) Slowly pour the melted wax into the hot oil, stirring constantly with a wooden spoon. If the oil is too cool, the wax will congeal like egg-drop soup, which actually is not a big concern. If this happens, simply keep the pan on the heat and keep stirring until you have a clear, homogenous mixture.
5) Once the wax incorporates into the oil, immediately remove the salve from the heat and carefully fill the jars.

Use of a pan with a pouring spout or a pyrex beaker with a spout is recommended.

6) Clean your pans and utensils while they are still hot by swiftly wiping them with dry cotton rags or paper towels, before the residual salve or wax has a chance to congeal.

7) Allow the tins or jars to sit still until the salve hardens. Then put on the lids and store in a dark, dry, and cool place. Salve will melt if left in the sun. Salve has an expected shelf-life of 2 years.

Note: Adding a slightly higher ratio of wax to oil will result in a salve of harder consistency, which will hold up better in warm weather. In therapy, harder salves (more wax) have a protective influence, while softer salves (less wax) allow for better absorbency of the herbal principles. For example, lip balm is best made with a high percentage of wax in order to form a thick layer that shields the lips from sun and wind. A healing salve is made intentionally soft so that the herbs can better penetrate the injured tissues.

Example 2: Healing salve

Formula (infused oil): 1:5 (dry herb weight in g:oil volume in ml)
Formula (salve): 100:17 (vol. herbal oil in ml:weight beeswax in g)

100 g comfrey dried roots
50 g calendula dried flowers
50 g goldenseal dried leaf
50 g plantain dried leaf
1250 ml olive oil to yield 1000 ml oil after pressing and filtering
170 g beeswax pieces, melted

This salve is useful for treating shallow cuts, scrapes, chapped skin, diaper rash, etc.

Procedure for making healing salve:

In this case, instead of extracting the herbs individually and then combining the oils, the dried herbs are combined together prior to adding the oil and are then digested together. This produces a compound oil, which contains the extractives from these several herbs. This oil is then further used to make salve according to the general formula and procedure for making herbal salve.

Basic Formula for Skin Creams
1:3:1
(wax in g: herbal oil in ml:distilled water in ml)

Example: Medicated cream

A handful of fresh flowers
50 ml distilled water
150 ml oil (olive, almond, jojoba, or sesame) or the same quantity of an infused herbal oil such as calendula oil, figwort oil, etc.
50 g beeswax pieces
1 Vitamin E 1000 I.U. perle (10 drops)
30 drops (more or less) essential oils of choice—optional

This cream provides a moisturizing, cleansing, and cooling effect, with healing attributes depending on the properties of the fresh flowers, herbal oils, and essential oils being used.

General procedure for making skin creams:

1) Bring the water to boil in a saucepan.
2) Add fresh flowers of choice (e.g. borage flowers, cowslip flowers, marigold petals, or marshmallow flowers). Cover and let the flowers steep until cool.
3) Strain through several layers of cheesecloth and collect the flower water in a bowl. You may squeeze the flowers in the cheesecloth to express the last bit of liquid. Pour the flower water back into a saucepan, put on a lid, and set it aside.
4) In a double boiler, melt the beeswax. For a thin cream, use less wax. For a robust cream, use more wax.
5) Add the oil to the beeswax. For a very mild cream, use straight olive, almond, jojoba, or sesame oil. For a more strongly medicated cream, use an infused herbal oil such as arnica, calendula, or Saint John's wort oil. Keep the double boiler on the heat and stir the beeswax and oil together until they incorporate completely.
6) Stir in the Vitamin E oil (squeeze it out of the perle).
7) Heat the flower water until it attains approximately the same temperature as the wax-oil mixture (both should read about 158° F (70° C)).

8) Remove your pan of oil and beeswax from the double boiler and away from the heat. Using a hand or electric mixer, begin beating the oil-wax mixture and have some-one slowly dribble in the flower water, 1 tablespoon at a time, while you continue beating, until emulsification is complete (about 10 minutes). You can also use a blender for this process. Emulsification is a process wherein a watery substance is dispersed and suspended in an oily substance. The clear oil-wax mixture will turn white and harden into cream. The key to successful cream making is to add the flower water *very* slowly.

9) Thoroughly stir in the essential oils at the starting rate of 1 to 2 drops per oz. Use greater or lesser quantities of essential oils depending on the relative strength or mildness desired. A few examples of essential oils to use include: lavender, rose, rose geranium, and rosemary.

10) Scoop the cream into sterile, wide-mouth jars. Using a clean cloth, wipe the rims free of any drips, and then screw on the lids. Label appropriately. Store in a dark, dry, and cool place. If stored in the sun, melting and separation are likely to occur. Herbal creams made in this manner require no additional preservatives and have an expected shelf-life of 6 months to 1 year.

Chapter 11
Poultices, Compresses, and Soaks

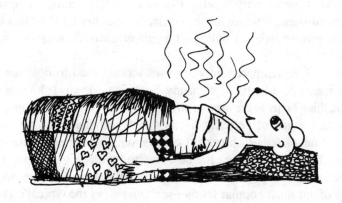

Midwinter found us huddled in our eight-sided wooden yurt that was set up in the middle of the fallow, wind-swept garden. We could gaze out the windows at a wide view of Grayback Mountain where it presided over brown fields and treed slopes from under a mantle of heavy snow. We had both our wood cookstove and a wood-fired heating stove set up in the uninsulated structure and had filled the gaping cracks between the wall boards and the roof with raw sheep's wool. We even filled every knothole in every board with a plug of wool, but still the cold seeped through. It was standard practice to put knitted caps on all the kids before bedtime. This particular night, the two older ones had climbed up into the sleeping loft, while Mayche and I bedded down with Sena, our four-year-old blonde-headed wisp, on a futon mat on the floor. I lay awake for a while, entertained by the sound of the wind that dropped down from the mountain and swirled around the yurt. I remember thinking, "If we had shutters, they'd be shakin' now!" Then, wishing we *did* have shutters on the windows, I drifted off.

Somewhere around the middle of the night, Mayche shook me awake. "Sena can't breathe," she said. I could see in the bare moon and starlight that the little girl's shoulders lifted with each breath, breaths that came hard and rattled in her throat. It is like that with kids sometimes—upper respiratory infection can flare up in a few hours, and then can disappear almost as quickly under the right care. But this was frightening. Mayche soothed Sena, holding her in her lap and gathering the blankets close around, while I pulled on a pair of pants, lit a candle, and tried to think.

I remembered how my own mother used to hold me in the steam of a kettle to clear my breathing. Then, I thought of something better in the form of an onion poultice. This is a compound poultice made of partially fried onions, cornmeal, and vinegar, and it never fails to break up congestion. I was used to making them because they were the best way to treat Jeb's recurring ear infections. But this was a poor household, and as onions were one of our most popular foods—making savory the typical diet of brown rice, tofu, and kale—we happened to be completely out of them at the moment. In a desperate stretch of recollection, I flashed on the previous day when I had traversed the frozen garden and nearly stepped on an oblong onion, for some reason rejected or forgotten during fall harvest.

Mayche said, "Hurry up and do something." In seconds I was out the door and in the garden. The wan moonlight and the desperate energy of necessity guided my bare feet to the onion. It was half-buried and yielded to my fingers like a partially frozen placental blob, but I squeezed out a core of good onion—just big enough for a small poultice.

There was a gas burner set up in the tiny porch, and I danced around on freezing feet finding the right utensils. I lit the fire, put on an iron skillet, found the cutting board and knife, and finely minced the onion. Then, dribbling a little olive oil in the pan, I put in the onion pieces and stirred them around with the knife. I had to go inside to find the vinegar and the cornmeal. Sena was gulping for air and Mayche was rubbing her chest and back, coaching each breath. She gave me a telling glance that sent me hurrying back out to the porch. The onion was just right, about half-fried, so I poured in a generous cup of vinegar, which bubbled and fumed. Then I threw in a few scant handfuls of cornmeal, and stirred the ingredients to a stiff paste. Draping a clean diaper over a plate, I scraped the steaming mush on top, spread it about an inch thick, and made my way back to the bed. We laid Sena back and bared her chest. After ascertaining that it was not too hot, I slid the moist, gooey cloth gently onto her upper chest and throat, tucked the edges of the diaper under her armpits, and covered the poultice first with a plastic bag and then with a towel and a blanket.

We sat back on our heels to watch. The alliaceous and vinegar-laden fumes rose up, making our eyes smart and having a clearing effect even on *our* breathing. Sena also took an easier breath, then swallowed and took several more breaths, each deeper than the last. She never had been fully awake as far as we could tell and, within a few more breaths, she developed a dreamy expression and settled in.

My wife and I exchanged glances while the adrenaline slid out of our systems and our hearts quit thumping. Then in unison, we shrugged our shoulders and cuddled back in on either side of the sleeping child. More sleep was a welcome prospect.

I went up on one elbow and hardly had the strength to blow out the candle. We awoke to full morning light, and I rolled over immediately to check on Sena. Her eyes were open, pretty as bluebells, staring at the rough boards of the ceiling. When she saw me, she smiled. "Daddy," she said, "can I have another one of those?"

* * * * * * *

Poulticing is well-understood by native peoples, but modern practitioners, even many herbalists, largely ignore the technique. During my high-school days, I had the opportunity to do some archaeological survey work in the Sierra Nevada of Colombia. My lanky, black-bearded work partner, Jack, was walking on the white sand beach near Santa Marta and stepped on something sharp. We washed the wound with soap and water, put on a light bandage, and didn't think much more about it. The next day we woke up early, because we planned to head up into the mountains. Rounding up our crew of three locals, we packed enough food for a few days, sharpened our machetes, and eventually rode out. One of my stirrups immediately broke off the strap. José, a chubby-faced youth with a perennial smile flashing out from under a squished, white cowboy hat, bound the stirrup back to the strap using what looked like kite string. After that, I put less pressure on the stirrups.

By noon we were far above the settlements on a winding path that, at times, overlooked the blue-green coral reefs far below, but eventually plunged back into true jungle, a jungle thick with viny underbrush and crisscrossed with tinkling streams. As the trail disappeared into steaming, mosquito-ridden brush, we found it easier to ride in the shallow streams, using them as pathways to locate and survey the remains of the pre-contact Tairona settlements that were scattered everywhere.

We found several flat places where rounded, white foundation stones marked previous settlements or where giant, carven stone blocks were cleverly set to bridge the stream. In one place, stones formed a stairway leading up a hillside that was now completely overgrown and inaccessible.[12]

We made maps and collected representative samples of the pottery and ground stone tools that eroded from the stream banks. The collection bags, bulging with potsherds, weighed heavily on the horses and, due to this increased load, we now led them instead of riding. Their hooves clacked against the streambed, accompanied by the sound of the pottery clinking and grinding and by the occasional twang of machete on vine. Giant toads lay still among the rocks of the streams. These we avoided, as they were reportedly poisonous and were definitely very, very ugly.

On the second night out, we bivouacked in an empty, thatch-roofed cabin situated on top of a knoll that afforded a little relief from the sun, the still air, and the mosquitoes. We peeled and boiled a few starchy yucca roots (*Manihot esculenta*) and hungrily ate these, along with some soup, for our communal

---

[12]I still have a recurring dream of walking (or floating) up these steps, with the azure and emerald jungle parting before me. At the top I find an ancient garden, redolent with perfumes of flowers which I know are extinct, pendulous red-fringed corollas giving way to toothsome fruits . . .

supper. As the firewater (*agua diente*) went around and before the Colombians got involved in their usual inexplicably exciting game of dominoes, Jack commented that his foot was feeling worse. He lay back on a hammock and we all gathered about, pulling off first his boot and then his sock. There was an angry, red slice in the sole of his foot and after one glimpse of the growing infection, our one-armed guide, Don Luis Calbo, went purposefully off into the darkening jungle. He returned shortly with a single, smooth, green leaf. Adeptly using his one hand, he applied a small amount of lard to the leaf and warmed it on the glass chimney of the oil lamp, working it back and forth until the lard had melted and the leaf turned warm and flexible. Then, without bathing or cleaning the wound in any way, he applied the leaf to the injured foot, repeatedly smoothing it to the area around the infected wound. We then replaced the sock, thereby holding the leaf in place, and Don Luis told Jack not to walk on the foot until morning.

The night progressed slowly and wakefully, as is always the case when one is trying to make a cheap Colombian hammock into a bed. I imagined the scurrying of giant cockroaches below my swinging, banana-shaped form. There was only one real disturbance, caused when a rat climbed into Jose's hammock and began gnawing on his uncured leather belt. "Rato'n, rato'n!" he cried, flinging the rat away from him. It thumped down somewhere in the darkness, while the rest of us snickered unsympathetically from our hammocks.

The red morning sun finally arose, accompanied by the far-off howling of a monkey troupe and the raucous cries of flapping hordes of varicolored birds. The Colombians were up, cooking the inevitable oatmeal and harrying a midsized python that had taken up residence in the thatched roof of the hut. Jack moaned, and I gratefully swung out of my torturous hammock. Remembering the little scurrying noises of the night before, I carefully shook out my boots before pulling them on and lacing them up. I rubbed my eyes, observing that Jack was still reclining. Taking pity on him and mumbling a few words of explanation, I removed his sock and then rubbed my eyes again in disbelief. There, on the *outside* of the leaf, was a glob of white, purulent matter that had been sucked from his wound. Upon removing the leaf, I had another surprise. The cut, now shrunken, less red, and apparently on the way to healing, had given up a treasure. There was a perfect little snail shell resting between the lips of the cut, probably introduced on the beach soon after the cut was made and sucked from deep inside the tissues by Don Luis' poultice. Using the tweezers from my Swiss army knife, I plucked up the shell and dropped it into Jack's outstretched palm, a mother-of-pearl gem gleaming in the morning light. Such is the power of a single leaf.

Poultices

A poultice is simply vegetable material, whole or mashed, which is layered or spread on the skin. Its primary function is to pull poisonous or infected matter from swollen tissues, wounds, or cysts. The hot poultice (maximum 105° F = 41° C) increases circulation, while the cold poultice reduces inflammation. Poultices also permeate the injured area with healing substances from the plant. A poultice is the herbal equivalent of "laying on hands," but in this case it is "laying on leaves."

Certainly the simplest technique of poulticing is to chew a leaf and spit it onto the affected part. A more sanitary approach is to wrap the injured area in fresh leaves, a procedure which, if conscientiously and repeatedly performed, can be effective treatment for afflictions ranging from an infected cut to rampant gangrene. Almost any green leaf from a broadleaf tree or plant will do, as long as one avoids overtly spiny, hairy, poisonous, or acrid plants. I have had good success using blue vervain, chickweed, dandelion, dock, English ivy, figwort, jewelweed, marshmallow, mullein, and plantain for poulticing.

In order for a poultice to do its work, it must be adhered to the skin. Thin, smooth leaves (e.g. dandelion and plantain) may be bruised and moistened with their own juice, placed in layers to the skin, tied in place with strip of cotton cloth, and then left for several hours (or preferably overnight) to do their work. Thicker or fuzzier leaves (e.g. marshmallow and mullein) need to be lightly steamed until flexible and then applied hot. Apply towels for insulation before wrapping with a long strip of cotton cloth, which is then tied in place.

Example 1: Comfrey poultice

Procedure dry root:

1) Use the dried roots of comfrey, ground up as finely as possible.
2) The quantity used is dependent on the area of coverage desired. A midsized poultice will require about 100 g of dried root.
3) Moisten the root powder with sufficient hot water to make a stiff paste.
4) Spread the paste directly on the injured area to a thickness of approximately 1 inch (2.54 cm).
5) Cover the area with a clean cotton cloth.

The poultice is preferably applied last thing before bed, left on all night, then scraped away and washed off in the morning. If the poultice is to be applied during the day, it may be secured with a long strip of cotton cloth. Repeat the procedure several times daily until the affliction is cured. Comfrey poultices are excellent for repairing traumatic damage to bones, tendons, muscles, nerves, or spinal cord. Comfrey causes rapid cell proliferation, helps dissolve and remove dead tissue, and markedly speeds healing.

Note: Comfrey poultices are not recommended for use on deep, infected wounds or puncture wounds, because they promote quick healing of the surface tissues, which can trap infection in deeper tissues. In the case of puncture wounds, Epsom salt therapy is a better approach (see "Epsom Salts Soak," pages 101–102).

Procedure fresh whole plant:

1) Dig the fresh roots and very thoroughly scrub them with a scrub brush, to remove the black, slimy cortex.
2) Chop up the roots with an equal portion of fresh, green comfrey leaf and combine these in a blender, using only sufficient water to cause the mucilaginous goo to vortex.
3) Spread the fresh paste directly on the injured area and cover with a clean cloth. Further directions as per dry root procedure, above.

Example 2: Flaxseed poultice formula

Formula: 1:3 (ground flaxseed in g:water in ml)

Procedure:

1) Grind 30 g (~1 oz.) of flaxseed to a powder and add to 90 ml cold water, stirring continually.
2) Spread the paste evenly over the injured area—cover first with a layer of plastic and then with a towel.
3) If mobility is desired, cover first with plastic, then a light cotton cloth secured with a cotton strip.

Flax is the quintessential drawing herb, making an excellent poultice for drawing out pain, swelling, splinters, infection, or poisons. Grind seeds only as needed, using an electric coffee mill.

* * * * * * *

A woman came to me, asking for help with an injured knee. "I fell with all my weight on this knee—it hurt like crazy and started to swell. I put ice on it, and the doctor told me to keep up with the ice and take these anti-inflammatory pills." "How long ago was that?" I asked. "Over a month," she answered, and lifted up her pants leg. The knee was boggy with retained fluids, dead white, and when I cupped my hand over it, felt completely cold.

"Well," I said, "It looks like there is stuck fluid around the knee, and even though the injury was some time ago, I'd still recommend using arnica oil. Soak a washcloth in hot epsom salt water and hold it to the knee, repeatedly wringing out the cloth and reapplying. Do this for about 20 minutes. Then, dry the knee and rub in the arnica oil." "How often should I do this?" she asked, and I answered, "Two or three times a day. And by the way, discontinue the ice and the pills."

Two days later I saw her again. "It's working, but now it hurts!" she said, and pulled up the pants leg. I could see that the swelling was way down, and the knee felt warm, but the tiny miracle was this—under the gentle influence of arnica oil and Epsom salts, the long repressed bruise had finally appeared, a blue-purple halo of healing surrounding her living kneecap.

Compresses

The compress (fomentation) is simply a cotton cloth soaked in dilute tincture, full-strength infused herbal oil, castor oil, herbal tea, or decoction that is applied to the skin and held in place by hand or by a long strip of cotton cloth. The compress may be renewed again and again by soaking in the herbal extract. This therapy is quite effective for treating localized afflictions of the skin, muscles, tendons, joints, and throat.

Example 1: Arnica tincture compress

Procedure:

1) Pour 1 cup (240 ml) of cold water into a ceramic or glass bowl.
2) Add the 2 droppersful (60 drops) arnica tincture, and stir.
3) Soak a light cotton cloth in the diluted tincture and place over the bruised, swollen, or painful part.
4) Renew every few minutes. Continue therapy several times daily to reduce pain and swelling, until the area is healed.

Arnica compresses are best used on unbroken skin, for treating athletic or other traumatic injuries. This compress is a specific remedy for dispelling bruises and alleviating swelling.

Example 2: Saint John's wort oil compress

Procedure:

The infused oil of Saint John's wort is used full-strength. Soak a light cotton cloth in the oil and place over the injured area, securing with a long strip of cotton cloth. The compress may be renewed periodically by resoaking in Saint John's wort oil. For deep wounds or infections, alternate with Epsom salt soaks. After soaking, dry the skin surface with a clean cloth and reapply the oil. Continue the therapy until the damaged tissues are healed. This compress may be used on broken or unbroken skin, for treating damaged nerve tissue, sore muscles, or other traumatic injuries.

Herbal Soaks and Baths

Because a soak or a bath involves a large volume of water and because absorption of herbs through the skin is not necessarily very efficient, you have to use a lot of herbs to get the desired effect. The entire body can be treated by soaking only the hands and feet, as circulation is stimulated by the hot water while the herbs are picked up and distributed throughout the system. Or, you can immerse yourself completely, which works wonders.

Basic procedure for herbal soaks and baths:

Make a quart (~1 L) or more of very strong tea or strong decoction, strain, and add it to the hot bath or soak. The maximum temperature for a hot bath or soak should be 105° F, which is equivalent to 41° C. Keep soaking for up to 20 minutes, then lie in bed and rest. Repeat up to 3 times per week.

Example 1: Rosemary bath

Procedure:

Make 2 quarts (~2 L) of a strong infusion of dried rosemary leaves, strain, and add to a full hot bath. To augment the effects, 4 cups of Epsom salts may also be added (see next page). Soak for 15 to 20 minutes. The vascular system will be stimulated, but the body must still rest. Wrap in a cotton sheet and go to bed, tucked in well with blankets. You will sweat. After a few minutes, replace the wet sheet with a dry sheet and stay in bed for at least another hour. The bath may be repeated up to 3 times per week. In place of the rosemary infusion, 1 dropperful (~30 drops) of rosemary essential oil can be used in the bath, but the whole herb is really superior.

A lavender bath may be made in exactly the same manner, but the effects are a little different. Lavender is more calming to the nerves, and less stimulating to the circulation.

Example 2: Witch hazel sitz bath

Procedure:

In a sitz bath, the quantity of liquid is kept to a minimum in order to increase the concentration of herbs. Make a quart (~1 L) of strong decoction of dried witch hazel leaves and pour this into 1 or 2 gallons of tepid water in the bottom of a small tub. Sit in it for at least 20 minutes. You will look ridiculous, and feel vastly relieved. Containing up to 9% tannins, witch hazel is a very efficient astringent and, as such, shrinks swollen tissues, reduces pain, and speeds healing. The witch hazel sitz bath is a specific treatment for postpartum trauma, perineal stitches, or hemorrhoids. If there is any potential for infection, 1 tablespoon (15 ml) of calendula tincture or succus may be added. Continue the sitz baths as needed, as often as 3 times per day, until the area is healed.

Epsom Salts (Magnesium Sulfate) Soak
1:8
(Epsom salts in g:hot water in ml)

This is not an herb, but a natural mineral substance too effective to be ignored, altering the osmotic balance of the tissues, drawing out dirt and suppurating matter, and increasing circulation to the injured areas. Epsom salt soaks are the most useful treatment available for puncture wounds and are also good for treating septicemia (blood poisoning), slow-healing infections, pustules, wounds, open ulcerations, bed sores, aches and pains, and poor circulation.

Examples of typical dilutions:

1 cup Epsom salts in 2 quarts hot water or
250 g Epsom salts in 2 L hot water

Procedure for making an Epsom salt compress:

Mix Epsom salts into very hot water. The water temperature should not exceed 105° F = 41° C. Stir until the salt dissolves. Soak a clean cloth in the hot Epsom salt water, and wring it out so it will not drip. Repeatedly bathe the injured area with this hot compress, renewing as soon as it begins to get cold. Continue for at least 10 minutes. Allow the area to air-dry. The compress is best used when a small affliction is on an area of the body which is difficult to immerse, for instance a bed sore on the hip, an earache, a painful pimple on the cheek, a sore neck, or an infected insect bite on the shoulder.

Alternating hot and cold:

For treating sprains, tendonitis, pulled muscles, wrenched back, or athletic injuries, alternate hot epsom salt soak with ice packs, changing several times in the space of 20 minutes, and ending with ice.

Procedure for making an Epsom salt hand or foot soak:

Mix the Epsom salts in 1 gallon of very hot (not scalding) water in a large bowl or bucket and stir until it dissolves. The water temperature should not exceed 105° F = 41° C. Plunge your feet or hands into the water and hold them there for as long as can be tolerated, then plunge momentarily into a basin of cold water. Alternate between hot and cold plunges, gradually increasing the length of time in the Epsom salts. The hot-cold alternation further accentuates the circulatory stimulant effects of Epsom salts. The hand or foot soak is good for treating general circulation problems or specific afflictions of the hands or feet, such as a puncture wound or infected finger or toenail. If there is an infection, 1 tablespoon (15 ml) of calendula tincture or succus may be added, to increase the antimicrobial potential of the soak.

Epsom Salt Bath

The full Epsom salt bath is good for treating general aches and pains, soothing the nerves, and is even a good treatment for cancer patients, as it assists in the elimination of toxins through the skin. This bath stimulates general circulation and increases the heart rate.

Contraindications: Full immersion Epsom salt baths are not recommended for people suffering from hypertension or low red blood cell count.

Procedure:

Use at least 4 cups (1 kg) of Epsom salts per bath. Make the bath hot (maximum 105° F = 41° C). Dissolve the Epsom salts into the water, ease in, and stay there for 15 to 20 minutes. Towel dry and rest. Using this volume of Epsom salts may seem a little extravagant, but your body will thank you for it. Besides, after what you went through on this day, you deserve it!

Part 2

A Gardener's Herbal Formulary

A formulary is a kind of recipe book, a concise reference meant to outline the best forms of medicinal preparations to be made from a wide array of substances. This gardener's herbal formulary is organized as an alphabetical listing by common name of useful medicinal herbs that can be cultivated by gardeners in temperate climates, that is in areas that have cold winters, but also enjoy a reasonably long growing season. For the most part, if you can ripen tomatoes in your garden, you can grow these herbs to fruition. Some of the plants listed herein are easy cultigens (e.g. calendula, cayenne, oats, and spilanthes). Some are first class European medicinal herbs that are also pretty easy to grow (e.g. elecampane, marshmallow, motherwort, and rosemary). Others are wild weeds that may be commonly encountered pathside, whether put there on purpose or freely volunteering (e.g. chickweed, dandelion, plantain, and self-heal). Some are more elusive wild plants (e.g. arnica, ashitaba, echinacea, gentian, and goldenseal), that may take some effort to successfully culti-vate in the home garden. Lomatium and osha have only recently yielded to domestication, and are new to this formulary. Hooray! I have also included some of the main herbs from the Chinese tradition (e.g. astragalus, dang-shen, dang-gui, and ma-huang), and others from the Ayurvedic tradition (e.g. ashwagandha, brahmi, gotu kola, and tulsi—holy basil), all of which have become quite familiar to western herbalists. At this point, it is difficult to live without them! Many of the main medicinal trees are represented (e.g. chaste tree, cramp bark, hawthorn, juniper, linden, and slip-pery elm). All-in-all, this formulary reflects the great diversity of healing plants used worldwide. Knowing them, their individual nuances of plant part and preferred preparation, will help you know what to make with your harvest and lead you toward appro-priate usage, as well. This is local herbal medicine at its best—inexpensive, effective, empowering, and liberating!

The discussion under each listing includes recommendations on harvesting, processing, and the choice of plant part. A shorthand summary of the complete formula for each kind of extract (e.g. 1:2 (100A)) is given, and the reader is advised to refer back to "Part 1," (especially chapter 4, "Standard Tincturing Ratios," page 30–31) to learn how to interpret this shorthand. Before getting out the shovel, the knife, and the bottle of grain alcohol, it would make sense to review the procedural details of how to make your extract of choice. These details are included throughout "Part 1." However, these basic procedures do not always tell the whole story. Therefore, specific hints on special harvesting, processing, and medicine making techniques have been inserted throughout the formulary where needed. Also included are the practical uses, consisting of the known actions and indications for each herb, tempered by my own experience with using them for healing family, friends, and myself. For a detailed discussion of basic effective dosage and the definition of my oft-employed phrase "Dosage: according to basic recommendations," the reader is referred back to "Part 1, Chapters 5 through 9." These chapters contain information on determining the appropriate size and frequency of dosage based on the potency of the herb, the concentration of the extract, the urgency of the situation, and the age, size, and constitution of the patient. In "Part 2, A Gardener's Herbal Formulary," I have carefully listed individualized and specific dosage ranges for all low-dose botanicals. These must be handled with care and taken only under the advice of a qualified health professional. Finally, the information found under "Contraindications" is meant to provide relevant cautions, whether related to pregnancy, undesirable combinations or practices, dosage issues, time factors, potential for allergic reactions, or overt toxicity. I would ask the reader to carefully consider the advisability and appropriateness of using each herb:

An herb used carelessly can harm, while the same herb dispensed from knowing and loving hands will heal hurt and banish suffering.

Welcome to this practical formulary. I hope you prop this book up at the back of the counter and that it is soon stained with the happy splatter of utilization.

A

Aloe vera (True Aloe)
Family: Asphodel (*Asphodelaceae*)

Parts used: The mucilaginous gel contained in fresh, fleshy leaves. Once removed from the plant, this gel has a very short shelf-life, being subject to enzymatic, oxidative, and microbial degradation in storage. Popular products containing aloe gel or aloe juice must contain preservatives. Therefore, maximum purity and efficacy is achieved by using the fresh gel obtained from your own houseplants! There is really no advantage in trying to tincture *Aloe vera*, as the mucopolysaccharides (galactomannans) do not remain stable in an alcoholic base. The herb gives best results when applied from the plant directly to the skin, or ingested in the fresh state.

Preparation: For topical application of the mucopolysaccharide-rich gel, a large, basal leaf may be cut from the *Aloe vera* plant and squeezed so as to release the gel. This gel may be applied freely to damaged skin, as a moistening, cooling, and healing embrocation. To make a fresh leaf poultice, slice the leaf lengthwise to reveal the gel-filled interior, and apply the fillets gel-side-down, leaving on for 20 minutes. To prepare for internal use, cut the leaf from the plant and slice it lengthwise. Use a spoon to scrape the gel from the rind, and consume the gel as-is. If a laxative effect is desired, scrape deeply to the rind, including the yellow exudate, which is rich in the anthraquinone constituents aloin and aloe-emodin. If a laxative effect is not desired, scrape gently so as to exclude the majority of the anthraquinones, which reside mainly in a layer just below the rind.

Practical uses (topical): As a topical application, aloe gel treats all kinds of first- and second-degree burns including those caused by kitchen or industrial accidents, sunburn, radiation, and chemical burns. The sooner the gel is applied, the more effective it will be in cooling the burn, thereby curtailing skin damage. Thrice-daily applications will promote rapid healing, and may be continued until new skin has formed. The effect is cleansing, anti-inflammatory, antioxidant, antibacterial, and immune-enhancing. Aloe gel moistens the skin and speeds healing through increased fibroblastic activity, promoting rapid formation of granulation tissue. Other conditions that yield to external application of aloe gel include scrapes and other shallow wounds, age-related wrinkling and dryness, bacterial and fungal infections, dermatitis, psoriasis, genital herpes, skin ulcers, acne, frostbite, and poison oak/ivy. Apply the fresh gel to the affected area and continue this therapy until healing is complete.

Practical uses (internal): *Aloe vera* gel contains over 75 nutritive and medicinally active compounds, including vitamins, enzymes, minerals, galacto-mannans, anthraquinones, lignin, saponins, salicylic acid and 7 of the 8 amino acids required for good human nutrition. Taken internally, aloe gel provides a myriad of benefits. It soothes the oral and gastrointestinal mucosa, speeds healing of ulcerations and reduces inflammation, being an effective treatment for ulcerative colitis and acid reflux. Internal consumption of aloe gel helps rid the body of pinworms and threadworms. Aloe gel (as a carrier for the yellow anthraquinone known as aloin) has a laxative effect, softening stools and speeding peristalsis. It is a good treatment for constipation, and helps dispel toxins from the body. Aloe gel nourishes and promotes the immune-enhancing activity of the mast cells that reside in the body's connective tissue and especially mucous membranes, resulting in better overall immunity—an increased resistance to a wide array of pathogens. Aloin helps deactivate viruses, including those involved in herpes simplex and influenza. Antiseptic agents within the gel inhibit infections caused by fungi, bacteria, and viruses. Aloe is considered to be one of the most important anticancer herbs, exhibiting antineoplastic properties based on a combination of antiproliferative, immuno-stimulatory and antioxidant activities.

Dosage: External application as needed, 3 or more times daily until healing is accomplished. Internal dosage of fresh gel: 1 tablespoon up to 3 times daily until healing is accomplished.

Contraindications: External applications are well-tolerated by most users, including infants, children and adults. Rarely, if there is pre-existing sensitivity to plants in the lily family, allergenic reactions may occur. Internal use of aloe gel should be avoided by pregnant or nursing mothers, due to the possibility of uteral stimulation or passing the laxative effect on to the child.

Aloe vera x *vera*: In antiquity, wild stands of *Aloe vera* grew luxuriously along the upper Nile River in the Sudan. The special attributes of this aloe have long been recognized and greatly appreciated. For instance, Cleopatra purportedly used aloe gel as part of her daily beauty regime. Like all wild populations of species *Aloe*, the original plants were genetically diverse and capable of sexual replication by way of seed. However, over time, the original stands of *Aloe vera* were extirpated, and since then the plant has been maintained only in domestic culture, increased clonally by dividing the offshoots, the "pups." *Aloe vera* became very well-known and much utilized, but over time the capacity for reproduction by seed was lost. Most plants could be traced back to a single parent, and such clones are not mutually fertile. My interest in species *Aloe* led to an investigation of *Aloe vera*, and I discovered that both a yellow-flowered type and an orange-flowered type exist. Wouldn't it be possible to cross-pollinate these 2 varieties and, as it were, inject variation and the capacity for sexual reproduction back into *Aloe vera*? Parent plants of both types were obtained and planted in close proximity, in the tropics. Eventually, they flowered in concert, and instead of the usual empty seed capsules found on *Aloe vera*, these seed heads were filled with seed that proved to be fertile. It seemed like a long, long holding of the breath until the seedling plants grew to a size where they could be properly characterized. In the end, this progeny proved to be fertile, open-pollinated *Aloe vera* which resemble in every way the clonal *Aloe vera* that is so familiar to gardeners throughout the world—spotted in white, rubbery of spine, filled with glorious gel. We named this plant "*Aloe vera* x *vera*," as it is for all practical purposes *Aloe vera* crossed with itself. We release this plant to the public domain. We now have the ability to grow *Aloe vera* from seed!

Other species:

Cape aloe (*Aloe ferox*) is armed with strong, sharp spines (*ferox* means "fierce" in Latin), but nonetheless contains healing mucilage much like *Aloe vera*, and boasts even higher concentrations of vitamins, minerals and amino acids than its peaceful counterpart. *Aloe ferox* is easily cultivated and is common in its South African home. Since its leaves are massive, and richly endowed with the anthraquinone constituents, cape aloe has been employed since antiquity for production of aloe concentrates. The aloe gel is milked from the leaves and slowly simmered in a large iron pot until all moisture is driven off, leaving a black, crystalline exudate. This crude substance may be laboratory processed to produce the pure yellow bitter laxative powder known as "aloes." Cape aloe is not the only source plant for production of this yellow powder, but it is the best.

Krantz aloe (*Aloe arborescens*) is also native to South Africa, commonly planted to make interlaced, living fences that tower up to 8 feet tall—a formidable barrier against the passage of man and beast. Like *Aloe vera,* this is a preferred species for production of aloe gel, but more importantly, the soft leaves with rubbery spines are traditionally taken internally for treating advanced stages of cancer. The taste is mildly bitter, but soothing. The effect is antiproliferative, immunostimulating and antioxidant. Various protocols for preparing and ingesting this plant have been proposed, but alterative effects are due to the power of the herb, not the processing! The following regimen may prove effective: Cut the whole, fresh leaf into 2-gram "servings" and take thrice daily, slowly chewed and swallowed, chased with half a glass of pure water. The first dose can be taken first thing in the morning, on an empty stomach. The second dose can be taken just before lunch. The last dose should be taken last thing before going to bed. There is really no single cure for cancer. However, taken as part of a multifaceted anti-cancer program that includes lifestyle changes and traditional or alternative treatments, *Aloe arborescens* therapy is worth considering. Cancer is a serious disease, and all who are compromised by it are well-advised to seek professional care.

Andrographis
(Kalmegh, Chuan-xin-lian, King of Bitters)
(*Andrographis paniculata*)
Family: Acanthus (*Acanthaceae*)

Parts used: Entire plant, including root, leaf, stems, and flowers, used fresh or dried. Even the seedlings are shudderingly bitter, so one need not wait too long to make the medicine.

Tincture of fresh herb (preferred over dry): 1:2 (75A:25W)

Tincture of dry herb: 1:5 (50A:50W)

Water extracts: Tea made by infusing ½ teaspoon of the dried herb in 1 cup of hot water.

Succus of fresh leaves and stems: 1 part alcohol by vol.:3 parts andrographis juice by vol. (see "Chapter 9, Herbal Succi and Syrups," pages 74–75). The succus is a low-alcohol extract that may be used in ½ teaspoonful or less dosage, diluted in a little pure water or licorice tea, taken prior to eating, to stimulate appetite, reduce gas, and improve regularity of the bowels.

Practical uses: For treatment of poor liver function, the herb is both hepatoprotective and stimulating to the liver and bile secretion. Andrographis promotes digestion, cleanses the blood, and helps dispel toxins. For treatment of diseases involving blood spirochetes (e.g. malaria and lyme), the herb cools fevers and discourages or kills the pathogen. For treatment of colds, influenza, diarrhea, and dysentery, the herb is effective in ameliorating symptoms, arresting disease, and normalizing body function. Andrographis has a vascular-cleansing effect and has been used in treating heart disease (helping prevent buildup of fatty plaque in arteries) and thrombo-phlebitis (anti-clotting effect). The herb will help expunge intestinal worms. Andrographis is sometimes utilized in anticancer therapy, where it may prove to be anti-carcinogenic, anti-inflammatory, pain-relieving, and eliminative.

Dosage: Andrographis is intensely bitter, will exert its influence at low dosage, and may prove intolerable at higher dosage. A reasonable beginning dosage is 5 drops of the tincture or ⅓ cup of tea, taken 3 times daily just before meals. If well-tolerated, dosage may be increased over a few days time to 15 drops of the tincture or 1 cup of tea, 3 times daily. Child's dosage (age 6 and up): 1 drop of tincture or succus in licorice tea, taken up to 3 times daily, increasing to 3 drops if well-tolerated. If side effects (upset stomach or nausea) are experienced, reduce dosage until tolerable. Combining with good-tasting, antispasmodic and carminative herbs such as anise, fennel, licorice or cardamom is recommended, as this increases compliance and reduces side-effects.

Contraindications: Not to be used during pregnancy, lactation, or if trying to become pregnant. Andrographis may potentiate the effects of blood-thinning pharmaceuticals (e.g. coumadin or warfarin) and should not be used concurrently. Not to be used by individuals suffering from stomach or duodenal ulcers.

Angelica (*Angelica archangelica*)
Family: Carrot (*Apiaceae*)

Parts used: Entire aerial parts of the plant harvested prior to flowering and used fresh or dried. Root harvested in the autumn of the plant's first year of growth and used fresh or dried. Seeds harvested at maturity and dried.

Tincture of fresh roots or aerial parts: 1:2 (75A:25W)

Tincture of dried roots (preferred over fresh): 1:5 (50A:50W)

Tincture of seed: 1:4 (75A:25W)
Seeds do not soak up much liquid. Therefore, the extract may be made a bit stronger (1:4 instead of the more standard 1:5). The seeds can be ground up or bruised, soaked overnight in the menstruum, then briefly blended the following day and macerated in the usual manner.

Water extracts: Basic tea of dried seeds or the fresh or dried aerial parts. Angelica seeds are easy to add into tea mixtures. Basic decoction of dried roots or seeds.

Honeyed stems: Use the immature flower stalk, or remove the leaves from the green leaf stems of young angelica plants and cut into lengths (short enough to lie flat in a small saucepan). Add honey and simmer according to directions found on page 80. Honeyed angelica stems impart a warming and strengthening influence to the digestive organs and upper respiratory tract.

Practical uses: Angelica is an aromatic bitter, best taken before meals to improve digestion and prevent constipation and flatulence. The herb is also a serviceable emmenagogue used to help initiate menstruation and a diaphoretic to promote sweating in order to break fevers. Angelica tea is a warming beverage that helps reduce nausea, sneezing, and coughs associated with colds and flu, also improving overall immunity. The herb is an anti-inflammatory for treating asthma and rheumatism.

Dosage: According to basic recommendations found under "Dosage of tinctures," page 49–52 and "Dosage of teas and decoctions," pages 70–71. Always take the tincture well-diluted in a full cup of water.

Contraindications: Not to be taken during pregnancy. Taking extracts of the fresh root may irritate mucous membranes of mouth, throat, and GI—therefore, the extract of the dried plant is preferred. Angelica extracts may cause skin photosensitivity in predisposed individuals, although the dosage that is required to initiate this reaction is generally far greater than the recommended therapeutic dose. Take care during harvest as exposure to the plant juices on sensitive skin areas followed by exposure to the sun may cause photosensitive dermatitis (redness and blistering) that is both painful and long-lived.

Other species: Although *Angelica archangelica* is the official plant, there are over 50 species in the *Angelica* genus occurring worldwide, most of which are used medicinally by local peoples. Several American angelicas can be cultivated and made into serviceable medicine. These include the tenacious and highly aromatic *A. hendersonii* from the beaches of the west coast, the higher elevation *A. arguta* and *A. pinnata* of the western mountains, and one of the most striking of angelicas found worldwide, the giant purple angelica (*A. atropurpurea*) occurring in moist places in the midwestern and eastern states. See "Ashitaba" and "Dang-gui."

Anise (*Pimpinella anisum*)
Family: Carrot (*Apiaceae*)

Part used: Seeds harvested at maturity or when nearly mature and slightly green, and dried.

Tincture of seed: 1:4 (75A:25W)
The seeds may be ground up or bruised, soaked overnight in the menstruum, then briefly blended the following day and macerated in the usual manner.

Water extracts: Basic tea or decoction.

Practical uses: Anise is an aromatic stimulant to digestion and an effective carminative to help relieve gas associated with indigestion. The herb is used as an expectorant to treat dry cough, an antispasmodic for infant colic and hiccup, and as a flavoring agent to improve the taste of beverages or other medicines. Anise also promotes production of milk in nursing mothers.

Dosage: According to basic recommendations found under "Dosage of tinctures," pages 49–52 and "Dosage of teas and decoctions," pages 70–71. The dosage for infants is 1 teaspoonful (5 ml) of the tea, as required.

Contraindications: Large amounts not to be used during pregnancy.

Arnica (*Arnica montana, A. chamissonis*)
Family: Aster (*Asteraceae*)

Parts used: Aerial parts, especially the flowers, harvested at full flowering stage and used fresh or dried. The root may be used, but given the difficulty in getting plants started, it generally makes sense to leave the roots intact in order to produce an ongoing yearly harvest of the aerial parts. The roots of wild plants should never be disrupted. The roots offer no significant therapeutic advantage over the rest of the plant.

Tincture of fresh aerial parts or flowers: 1:5 (75A:25W)

Tincture of dried aerial parts or flowers: 1:10 (50A:50W)

Practical uses: Low doses of arnica tincture are used internally as an anti-inflammatory for treating traumatic injury. The herb also reduces pain and bleeding during and after surgery, improves nerve force, stimulates weak circulation, helps arrest urinary incontinence, and helps reduce emotional trauma associated with physical accidents or emotional shock.

Dosage: This is a low-dose botanical. Adult dosage is 5 drops of tincture diluted in 1 full cup of water, taken up to 3 times per day until the problem is resolved. Not for long-term use.

Oil, salve, or cream: Make infused herbal oil of the dried aerial parts, especially the flowers. This can be used as-is or can be further processed into salve or cream (see "Chapter 10, Basic Formulas for Herbal Oils, Salves, and Creams," pages 85–90). These products are for external application as an anti-inflammatory and resolvent for reducing swelling and bruising caused by traumatic injury, pulled muscles or ligaments, and for treating arthritic joints. See story page 98.

External use: To make a compress, dilute 1 part by volume arnica tincture:5 parts by volume cold water. Apply a clean cloth soaked in this solution directly to the injured area, renewing again and again until the inflammation and pain have subsided. Arnica tincture can also be added to hand or foot soaks for treating generalized trauma or arthritis. See "Chapter 11, Poultices, Compresses, and Soaks," page 99–102.

Contraindications as below:

Internal: Not for use during pregnancy. Arnica extracts are commonly labeled "not for internal use." However, I have never seen a side effect from the internal use of the diluted tincture, and it is my opinion and experience that the benefits outweigh the risks. Excessive dosage or hypersensitivity may result in gastric irritation, burning, or even ulceration of the gastric mucosa. If these symptoms appear, immediately discontinue use.

External: Not to be used on open wounds or broken skin. May cause allergic dermatitis in sensitive individuals. If the arnica seems to be *causing* redness and swelling instead of *reducing* these symptoms, then discontinue use.

Other species: Meadow arnica (*Arnica chamissonis*) is an indigenous American species that can be grown successfully in low elevation gardens. This plant has been tested and is generally approved as a substitute for *A. montana,* which is the official European species. The mountains of the United States are richly endowed with other *Arnica* species, all of which can be cultivated successfully in high elevation gardens. These include *A. cordifolia, A. latifolia* and more than 20 other, less common species. Although there has been little comparative testing of the constituents derived from the other indigenous American species, these have been used interchangeably and safely in folk medicine with good success. All species of the *Arnica* genus seem to do about the same thing and have similar strength. By the way, this blanket acceptance does not extend to so-called "Mexican arnica" (*Heterotheca inuloides*), which is a common adulterant of true arnica, inferior to it, and not even a close relative.

Artemisia annua (Sweet Annie, Qing-hao)
Family: Aster (*Asteraceae*)

Parts used: The leaves and immature flowers without the woody stems, harvested in the summer and used fresh or dried.

Tincture of fresh herb: 1:2 (100A)

Tincture of dried herb: 1:5 (75A:25W)
The tincture owes its unique activity to a synergistic combination of sesquiterpene lactones (including artemisinin) and flavonoids. Both classes of compounds are alcohol-soluble.

Water extract: Basic tea of the dried herb.

Practical uses (TCM): Qing-hao is used as a tea for treating heatstroke, giving relief from symptoms including low fever, mild nausea, headache, and dizziness—also for ameliorating the alternating fevers and chills of malaria.

Practical uses (western herbal medicine): The tincture of *Artemisia annua,* or the tincture in combination with a concentrated extract of artemisinin (in tablet form), is used for treating malaria. The herb interrupts the life cycle of the malarial spirochete and results in a rapid clearance of parasites from the blood. *Artemisia annua* has also shown promise in treating leukemia and non-small-cell lung cancer. Under the care of a qualified

114

health practitioner, the most effective regimen involves using the tincture and concentrated artemisinin concurrently, taken as part of a holistic anticancer therapy, often involving other herbs and supplements, exercise, and special diet.

Dosage: The tea is made with 3 to 9 grams of the herb in 1 cup (240 ml) of water and taken over the coarse of 1 day. The recommended dosage of the tincture is 1 to 2 droppersful, taken 3 times daily. Artemisinin is available over the counter in 100 mg tablets. The recommended dosage is 900 to 1,200 mg per day, taken in 3 equal doses, with meals.

Contraindications: Not to be used during pregnancy or nursing. Overdose of *Artemisia annua* or artemisinin may result in diarrhea, cold extremities, ringing in the ears, headache, and/or tunnel vision. Artemisinin therapy is contraindicated during radiation.

Artichoke, Globe (*Cynara scolymus*)
Family: Aster (*Asteraceae*)

Parts used: The leaves harvested just prior to flowering and dried. The flower buds (the "chokes"), harvested while young and succulent. The mature seeds.

Tincture of dried leaf: 1:5 (50A:50W)

Tincture of dried seed: 1:3 (100A)

Water extract: Basic tea of the dried leaves.

Practical uses: The tincture or tea of artichoke leaves or seeds, and to a lesser extent the chokes eaten as a nutritious food, are a valuable stimulant to the liver and the gall bladder, promoting production of bile and assisting in digestion of fats. The herb is a specific for treating dyspepsia caused by overeating or the excessive use of fats in the diet. The seed tincture demonstrates hepatoprotective activity (much like milk thistle, which see). Use of artichoke is a valuable therapy for treating arteriosclerosis, gallstones, elevated blood cholesterol, and obesity.

Dosage: According to basic recommendations found under "Dosage of tinctures," pages 49–52 and "Dosage of teas and decoctions," pages 70–71.

Food use: Thoroughly boil or steam the flower bud for 20 minutes or more, until the fleshy sepals (scales) are cooked through. Dip the scales in garlic oil or melted butter with garlic, and use the teeth to strip off the edible, fleshy portion. This comes along with a good deal of fiber that scours the gastrointestinal tract of toxins. Eat the heart, but reject the pappus hairs and spiny parts.

Contraindications: None known. Safe for general use.

Other species: The genus *Cynara* contains 11 species, several of which have been used for food and medicine. Cardoon (*C. cardunculus*) and wild artichoke (*C. humilis*) are progenitors to the globe artichoke and medicinally interchangeable with it. The leaf stalks of these plants are boiled and eaten, or the small flowers are used as a substitute for rennet in cheese making. Members of the *Cynara* genus should not be confused with Jerusalem artichokes (*Helianthus tuberosus*), which are only distantly related and are medicinally dissimilar.

Ashitaba (*Angelica keiskei-koidzumi*)
Family: Carrot (*Apiaceae*)

Parts used: Leaf stem and leaf, harvested prior to flowering and used fresh or dried. The plant has a unique habit of dropping its oldest leaf prior to making a new one. Harvest the oldest leaf and stem for herbal use before it becomes withered. This encourages the plant to grow larger and make new leaves, providing the gardener with ashitaba herb on an ongoing basis. The root, trunk, and flowers/seeds are potentially active but not usually utilized in medicine. Much of the unique activity of ashitaba may be attributed to the yellow, aromatic ketone-rich sap that wells up out of the plant when it is injured, or when the stems are cut at harvest. This yellow pigment contains unique molecules known as chalcones. Chalcones are poorly soluble in water, so this tasty herb is best used as a fresh food. The plant may also be dried and powdered for direct consumption or tincturing.

Tincture of dried stem and leaf: 1:5 (100A) Harvest, cut into ½ inch pieces, dry on screens, then grind to a coarse, dark yellow-green powder before extraction.

Powder: Grind the dried leaves and stems to a fine powder and take 1 teaspoon up to 3 times per day, chased with water, juice, or milk. This powder also incorporates well into smoothies.

Water extract: Basic tea of finely-cut dried stem pieces and leaves. The tea is a pleasant, effective way to enjoy the herb. For a stronger experience, use a teaspoonful of ashitaba leaf and stem powder stirred into ⅓ cup of cold water. After the powder is moistened, fill the remainder of the cup with boiling water. Stir, sip, and enjoy—sludge and all.

Practical uses: The growing plant demonstrates an incredible life-force and vigor, and seems to impart these qualities to its medicine. Native to Hachijojima in Japan, ashitaba has been tra-ditionally used as a rejuvenating food for at least 5 centuries, endowing the inhabitants of this island with good health and long life. This chlorophyll-rich herb contains substantive concentra-tions of Vitamins K, B1, B6 and B12, E, and C as well as carotene, calcium, potassium, and protein. When consumed fresh, these assimilable nutrients are delivered along with a great deal of dietary fiber, which helps scour toxins out of the system. The herb has a normalizing influence on blood pressure, blood sugar, and high cholesterol. It helps repair nerve damage, cleanses the colon, and acts to detoxify the liver. Ashitaba is used in treating eczema and psoriasis, disorders of the gastroin-testinal system, hepatitis, cancer, anemia, and chronic fatigue. In-vivo tests have shown strong antibiotic activity against drug-resistant staphylococcus.

Dosage: According to basic recommendations found under "Dosage of tinctures," pages 49–52 and "Dosage of teas and decoctions," pages 70–71.

Food use: Choose young, succulent leaf stems and leaves and sever at the base of the plant or where they attach to the stem of the plant. The leaf stem may be consumed fresh, like celery, and the leaves may be used sparingly in salads. The stems may be candied, stir-fried, steamed, or used in soup, where they combine favorably with dandelions, green onions, and shiitake.

Contraindications: Occasionally, users report side effects from ashitaba, including itchy skin, rash, or headache. These symptoms may be caused by the rapid die-off of harmful organisms within the body, resulting in release of endotoxins and lipoproteins into the bloodstream. If such symptoms occur, reduce dosage to once per day, drink plenty of water or herbal tea, and symptoms should soon abate. Dandelion is a good adjunct herb to use with ashitaba, as it helps eliminate toxins through the urine.

Ashwagandha (*Withania somnifera*)
Family: Nightshade (*Solanaceae*)

Parts used: Roots of 1- or 2-year-old plants dug in the autumn just after first frost and dried. In Ayurveda, the fresh roots are sometimes boiled in milk, prior to drying, in order to leach out undesirable constituents. Fresh root and aerial parts for poulticing. Berries for curdling milk.

Tincture of the dried root: 1:5 (50A:50W); see page 45.

Water extracts: Basic tea or decoction of the dried root.

Practical uses: The root of ashwagandha is an energy building sexual tonic and aphrodisiac. It is used for treating sexual exhaustion, impotence, sexual dysfunction, infertility, or low sperm count. As a sedative to the nerves and an adaptogenic tonic, the root is also useful for treating tiredness, senility, lack of concentration, drug burnout, and headache. The berries are used as a substitute for rennet, to coagulate milk in cheese making.

Dosage: According to basic recommendations found under "Dosage of tinctures," pages 49–52, and "Dosage of teas and decoctions," pages 70–71.

Poultice: The fresh root and leaves can be pounded into a poultice, used for resolving pimples, carbuncles, and for healing skin ulcerations. The poultice is also an anti-inflammatory treatment for rheumatic joints.

Direct consumption: The powdered, dried root is taken with milk or mixed into foods as a nutritive, rejuvenating tonic. The adult dosage is 1 to 2 tablespoons (3 to 6 g) per day.

Contraindications: Ashwagandha root is listed in the western literature as, "Not to be used during pregnancy." However, Ayurvedic practitioners use it as a pregnancy *tonic* and, after pregnancy, as a galactagogue to increase production of milk. The act of drying ashwagandha roots serves to reduce any potential side effects. Therefore, the roots should always be dried before taking internally. The aerial parts of the plant contain potentially toxic compounds and should not be used internally.

Other species: There are over 20 other species of the *Withania* genus that occur in the dry parts of India, Africa, and the Mediterranean. These include *W. coagulens* and *W. simonii,* the roots of which are sometimes used interchangeably with those of *W. somnifera.* The berries of these and other species of *Withania* (e.g. *W. frutescens*) are used in India and North Africa for coagulating milk. *W. somnifera* itself has been extensively selected and domesticated from the wild form. In India, at least five different cultivars have been developed for increased root size and adaptation to different climates. The medicinal attributes of the wild plants and the domestic strains are quite similar, although local practitioners will adamantly exhort the attributes of their local varieties.

Astragalus (Huang-qi) (*Astragalus membranaceus*)
Family: Legume (*Fabaceae*)

Part used: Roots dug in the fall of the second or third year of growth and used fresh or dried.

Tincture of the dried root: The typical cold extraction process does not work very well for astragalus, due to the fact that the water-soluble polysaccharides are best extracted with hot water, not cold alcohol. The best method of tincturing is to make a strong decoction and preserve it by adding sufficient grain alcohol to bring the final absolute alcohol content to 20%.

Water extracts (preferred over the tincture): Basic tea or decoction of the fresh or dried root.

Direct consumption: The fresh roots can be dug, washed, and chewed. Tasty, but fibrous enough to weave a welcome mat.

119

Practical uses: Astragalus is an immune-stimulating, blood-building, and liver-protective herb for treating wasting illness, physical weakness, poor appetite, liver disease, or anemia. Astragalus is used for recovery from radiation and chemotherapy. The herb also helps build energy and increase athletic stamina.

Dosage: According to basic recommendations found under "Dosage of tinctures," pages 49–52 and "Dosage of teas and decoctions," pages 70–71.

Food use: The fresh or dried root pieces can be added to soups, simmered for at least 30 minutes, then removed prior to serving. Fresh astragalus root would make a sensible addition to the produce section of food stores worldwide, to be sold as a vegetable for making soup.

Contraindications: Although astragalus is completely safe for consumption, the principles of traditional Chinese medicine (TCM) recommend that the herb be used during wellness. Not to be used to treat high fever or inflammatory infections.

Other species: There are over 1,000 species of the *Astragalus* (milk vetch) genus found worldwide, many with medicinal applications, many others useless or overtly toxic when taken internally. *Astragalus membranaceus* and *A. mongholicus* are both used to make the traditional Chinese medicine known as huang-qi. They are official and preferred. *A. americanus* is a species of northern North America, the root of which is reportedly nontoxic, but makes an inferior substitute for huang-qi. In Northern China, several other species are found in the wild, including *A. chinensis, A. complanatus,* and *A. adsurgens.* The roots of these species make a poor substitute for huang-qi, as they are fairly low in polysaccharides, but their seeds are valued, used to make a liver-tonifying medicine known as sha-juan-ji-li.

Bergamot (Bee Balm, Oswego Tea)
(*Monarda fistulosa, M. citriodora,*
M. didyma, M. punctata)
Family: Mint (*Lamiaceae*)

Parts used: Leaves and flowers, picked during early flowering stage and used fresh or dried. The entire flowering stalks may be cut, bundled, hung to dry, then rubbed through a coarse screen to remove the sticks and break up the flowers and leaves.

Tincture of fresh herb: 1:2 (100A)

Tincture of dry herb: 1:4 (75A:25W)

Water extracts: Basic tea of fresh or dried herb.

Poultice: Grind fresh bergamot to a paste and use for treating wounds or rub into rheumatic joints.

Oil, salve, or cream: Make infused herbal oil of the dried flowering tops. This can be used as-is or may be further processed into salve or cream (see "Chapter 10, Basic Formulas for Herbal Oils, Salves, and Creams," pages 85–90). Oily preparations are most useful in treating wounds, rheumatic joints, or if rubbed nightly behind the ear, tinnitus.

Sunny honey: Pack a crock or jar with fresh flowering tops and cover in honey, allowing to steep for 2 weeks on a sunny windowsill. Then, press out over a bowl, using a cheesecloth, or press out in a tincture press. Discard the marc and bottle the honey. This may be taken by the teaspoonful as often as needed, to allay sore throat, cough, tonsillitis, and/or laryngitis.

Practical uses: The tincture or tea are powerfully antibacterial and may be used to treat infections. Common colds and sore throat may be allayed by taking the tea or tincture, or by inhaling the vapors from a pan of boiling water sprinkled with dried bergamot. Containing volatile constituents carvacrol, geraniol, and rosmarinic acid, the effect is antiseptic, anesthetic, and anxiolytic (anti-anxiety, calming to the nerves). One of the many

Native American uses is in husband-taming, where the wise wife casually sets a pan of lovely-smelling bergamot to the back of the stove, in order to improve the mood of a grouchy male. A more potent form of this therapy involves using a bundle of bergamot in the sweat lodge, dipped in water and shaken on the hot rocks. The rising steam is highly therapeutic.

The tincture or cooled tea are tonic to the female reproductive tract. Rubbed into the abdomen or taken internally, they will prove of assistance in regulating the menses and treating urinary tract infection, whether caused by bacteria or yeast.

The tincture, tea, infused oil, or salve may be applied externally to contusions, wounds, and rheumatic joints. The effect is rubefacient, antiseptic, and healing. To use the tincture, dilute 2 droppersful in 1 cup (240 ml) of water and make a fomentation (soak a clean cloth and apply repeatedly to the affected area). The herbal tea may be used as a full-strength fomentation.

Dosage: According to basic recommendations found under "Dosage of tinctures," pages 49–52 and "Dosage of teas and decoctions," pages 70–71.

Spice: The dried leaves may be ground to a coarse powder and used as a carminative spice in the tradition of Italian or Mexican cuisine.

Contraindications: During pregnancy, food use is fine, but internal use of tea and tincture should be avoided.

A note on species: *Monarda* is a genus represented by 20 species, of which the above-mentioned plants are the most commonly used in traditional western medicine. These plants, loosely, may be used interchangeably in herbal medicine, but they are not the same. Each has its own flower color, flavor, constituent structure, and distinct natural distribution. Lavender bergamot (*M fistulosa*) is pungent. Lemon bergamot (*M. citriodora*) has a strong citrus scent. Sweet leaf (*M. fistulosa* var. *menthaefolia*) is purple-flowered and savory. Oswego tea (*M.didyma*) is red-flowered and mellow, while yellow-dotted mint (*M. punctata*) is minty. They are all well-loved by both downy mildew and bees.

Bilberry (Blaeberry, Whortleberry, Fraughan)
(*Vaccinium myrtillus*)
Family: Heath (*Ericaceae*)

Parts used: Berries, collected in their prime, used fresh or dried. Leaves, collected during the growing season, used dried.

Syrup: To make bilberry syrup, follow the directions for "Syrup Made from Reduced Berries" on pages 78–79.

Glycerite of dried berries (excellent!): 1:5 (60 Gly:40W)

Water extracts: Basic tea of the dried leaves. The ground, dried berries can also be made into a basic tea or decoction.

Direct consumption: The raw or dried berries or unsweetened juice from the fresh berries may be taken as-is, a delicious and effective way to realize the benefits of the herb.

Practical uses: The unsweetened juice, tea, or decoction of the dried, ground berries treats infant diarrhea. The effect is anti-bacterial and constipating. The fresh berries, dried berries, syrup, glycerite, and tea are effective in treating vascular fragility (spider veins and varicosities), improving eyesight and night vision, and for treating macular degeneration. The leaves contain arbutin, and may be used in the same manner as uva ursi, to treat urinary tract infection.

Dosage: According to basic recommendations found under "Dosage of tinctures," pages 49–52 and "Dosage of teas and decoctions," pages 70–71.

Contraindications: None.

Other species: Vaccinium is a genus of 450 species, mainly sub-shrubs growing in boggy places or in the forest understory, often at elevation. Cranberry (*V. macrocarpon*) juice is a popular beverage that (when taken unsweetened), is good to help prevent or recover from urinary tract infection. Hikers in the Pacific Northwest are familiar with huckleberries, a tasty trailside snack that provides some of the same vascular and ocular benefits as bilberry. Red huckleberries are *V. parviflorum*, and blue huckleberries are appropriately named "*V. deliciosum*."

123

Black Cohosh (*Cimicifuga racemosa* syn. *Actaea racemosa*)
Family: Crowfoot (*Ranunculaceae*)

Parts used: Root and rhizome (the root) dug during dormancy and used fresh or dried.

Tincture of dried root: 1:5 (50A:50W)

Tincture of fresh root (preferred): 1:2 (75A:25W)

Water extract: Basic decoction of fresh or dried root.

Practical uses: Black cohosh is used for allaying symptoms related to premenstrual syndrome (PMS) and menopause. It is also of assistance in treating weak, irregular, or delayed menses. The herb is a specific for treating rheumatic pain and other dull, aching body pains, as well as tinnitus (ringing in the ears). It can have an antidepressant effect, especially for elevating heavy, dark, oppressive moods. Using the herb during the last trimester of pregnancy and during labor will help improve the regularity and force of contractions, also assisting in rapid postpartum recovery.

Dosage: According to basic recommendations found under "Dosage of tinctures," pages 49–52 and "Dosage of teas and decoctions," pages 70–71.

Contraindications: There is an ongoing debate concerning the appropriateness of using black cohosh during pregnancy. The concern arises that an herb used to encourage the onset of delayed menses might cause abortion if used during pregnancy. However, the actual effects of the herb are more in the realm of normalizing irregularities of function in the female reproductive tract. The decision of whether or not to use black cohosh during pregnancy should be made by a qualified practitioner who has the constitution and medical history of the patient firmly in mind.

Other species: There are 18 closely related species of the *Cimicifuga* genus found in Europe, North America, and Asia. Although several of these, including the western bugbane (*C. elata*), have been used interchangeably with black cohosh, given the quirky and potentially toxic nature of the crowfoot family in general, I do not see much reason to cultivate other species for medicine. Black cohosh is easily cultivated, has been exhaustively tested in order to prove its harmlessness as a medicine, and the other species offer no added advantage. Wild-harvested black cohosh root is often adulterated with the root of red baneberry (*Actaea rubra*). The flowers and fruits of black cohosh and baneberry are quite dissimilar, but the dormant roots are difficult to distinguish from each other. The adulteration of black cohosh with baneberry may well be the cause of the rare side effects reported for "black cohosh root." Given the potential toxicity of red baneberry, this adulteration is a further impetus to the movement, now in force, to replace wild-harvested black cohosh with cultivated material.

Black Seed (*Nigella sativa*)
Family: Crowfoot (*Ranunculaceae*)

Parts used: Dried seeds.

Tincture of seeds: 1:3 (75A:25W) Bruise the seeds by pounding in a mortar and pestle or by grinding briefly in a coffee mill. Soak overnight in the menstruum, then blend the following morning and macerate in the usual manner.

Infused oil: 1:3 (dry seed weight in g: oil in ml) Bruise the seed (as above), place in a crock pot, and stir in the oil. Use organic olive oil or (as is done extensively in Africa and India) coconut oil. Black seed withstands and requires more heat for extraction than leafy herbs. Set the temperature to 122° F (50° C) and stir at least twice daily. Digest in this manner for 5 days, then press out the hot, infused oil by hand through 4 layers of cheesecloth into a bowl, or (superior) use a tincture press. See page 86.

Powdered seed: For treating intestinal parasites, the powdered seeds may be placed on the tongue and washed down with milk (dairy or nut-derived). Use of the ground seed (as opposed to the tincture) carries the vermifugal qualities deeply into the gut. Adult dosage is 1 teaspoonful (2 g) twice daily. For children aged 6 to 12, ½ teaspoonful (1 g) twice daily. For children aged 2 to 5, ¼ teaspoon (½ g) twice daily. This therapy needs to be maintained for 3 days duration. When treating parasitic conditions, it works best to eat lightly (raw foods including pumpkin seeds and fresh carrots are recommended) and drink plenty of fresh water throughout the day. Adults combine each dose with 5 drops tincture of andrographis (2 drops for children aged 6 to 12, 1 drop for children aged 2 to 5). In the evening, eat as usual. After 3 days, adults may take a dose of rhubarb as a laxative or aloe vera as a laxative and antiparasitic. Children or the aged will respond better to stewed prunes. This will clear the gut. See "Rhubarb" and "Aloe vera."

Culinary uses: Whole seeds are often used in the culinary arts, stirred into foods, or used as a sprinkle. They are decoratively jet-black, naturally perfumed, and help preserve freshness in foods—a little goes a long way! Black seed makes a strangely tasty garnish when sprinkled on cookies or mixed into candies, is found in many a curry, and is often added to naan (the soft, leavened flatbread made famous in Indian cuisine). *Panch phoron* (Bengali 5-spice blend) is composed of equal parts seeds of cumin, black mustard, black seed, fennel, and fenugreek. The seeds are stir-fried (tempered) in hot oil until they pop, which releases their essence. *Panch phoron* spices up meat, poultry, and potato dishes, and is also used to flavor beans and lentils. The effect is warming to the digestion, improves absorption of nutrients, and reduces gas.

Practical uses: Much of the traditional usage and recent scientific studies involve the expeller-pressed fixed oil of the seeds, a product that is widely available in Africa, Arabia, and India. Once, while travelling in East Africa, I suffered from a tropical fungus which arose uninvited between my swimmer's fingers. Hurrying to the local apothecary, I purchased an ounce of black seed oil (*mafuta ya habat soda*) and rubbed it on even as I navigated the streets, past shops offering all kinds of native remedies, past the battered stop sign that hung, largely ignored, at the main intersection of town, eventually making my way back to Sharook's guest-house. After 3 days time, having used the entire bottle, the affliction disappeared. This was in the town of Wete on the northern tip of the island of Pemba in the Zanzibar archipelago. If you can find black seed oil there, surely you can get it almost anywhere!

The infused oil can be made at home, producing a product that has the same applications as the fixed oil—similarly effective, but somewhat less concentrated. Among more than a hundred other active constituents, *Nigella sativa* contains a high percentage of alcohol- and oil-soluble thymoquinone (molecular formula $C_{10}H_{12}O_2$) which provides strong antioxidant, analgesic, and anti-convulsant properties. Applied externally, oil of black seed is used for treating rashes, hives, beestings, spider bites, scorpion stings, fungal afflictions, skin ulcerations and discolorations, bed sores, leprous sores, pustular anomalies, and itches—also for rubbing into painful or arthritic joints. The oil eases pain, reduces swelling, and is strongly antibacterial, antiviral, and antifungal. It also has an antineoplastic effect, reducing the blood flow to cancerous tumors. Both oil and alcohol extracts have been used against colon and breast cancer.

Directly consumed in foods or taken as a tincture, black seed proves antiparasitic, anti-inflammatory, hepatoprotective, anti-convulsant, digestive, and helps reduce the deleterious effects of food allergies. It is used in treating influenza, sinusitis, cough, asthma, seizures, and autoimmune diseases including HIV/AIDS and lupus. Digestive disorders, including obesity and loss of appetite are often improved by administering black seed. The tincture can be used externally as well as internally, and may be rubbed on rheumatic joints. For treatment of asthma, massage into the back and chest. Chew black seeds along with other aromatic carminatives such as caraway, anise, coriander, and ginger for treatment of diarrhea, indigestion, and for improving bad breath. According to Abu Hurairah, the sunni narrator of hadith, *"There is healing in black seed for all diseases except death."*

Dosage: According to basic recommendations found under "Dosage of tinctures," pages 49–52.

Contraindications: Not to be used during pregnancy (stimulates uterine contraction). Seeds toxic to invertebrates and fish.

Other species: Love-in-the-mist (*Nigella damascena*) bears jet-black, naturally perfumed seeds that may be used in cookies and confections. However, for the purpose of making medicinal tinctures and oils, purists insist on using black seed (*N. sativa*).

Bloodroot (*Sanguinaria canadensis*)
Family: Poppy (*Papaveraceae*)

Part used: The entire rhizome (the root) dug during dormancy or in the early spring when the plant is in flower, which is the stage of highest root sanguinarine content. The root is used fresh or dried.

Acetous extract: 1:10 (50A:50ACV)

Practical uses: The well-diluted tincture of bloodroot is used as an expectorant to relieve harsh, dry cough and help thin and expel mucous. The root is applied full-strength externally against abnormal skin growths. Diluted and taken orally, bloodroot sometimes demonstrates an antitumor effect. This may be due to the presence of the antimitotic alkaloid known as sanguinarine, or it may be due to the fact that the herb helps free up and disperse toxins, a property that is generally shared by acrid herbs. In the end analysis, it may be found that the antitumor effects are actually due to a combination of both factors.

Dosage: This is a low-dose botanical, best used under the care of a qualified health care professional. Adult dosage is 5 drops diluted in a cup of cold water taken 3 to 5 times daily. Not for long-term usage. If taken internally, it is best to combine bloodroot with emollient, antiseptic, and immune-enhancing herbs (e.g. mullein, elecampane, and marshmallow) to protect the mucous membranes and for a more rounded effect in treating upper respiratory infection.

External use: The dilute tincture is not very useful for external application. However, the sliced root can be quite effective when rubbed on ringworm or warts. This treatment must be repeated at least twice daily, allowing the bloodroot juice to dry on the spot. Ringworm usually disappears in 2 or 3 days. Warts may take up to 2 weeks to fall off. Localized inflammation during this therapy is simply an indication that the herb is doing its work and should not be considered to be a dangerous side effect. This treatment is not effective for plantar warts (deeply embedded warts on the sole of the foot).

Bloodroot salve: The powdered, dried bloodroot is mixed into a sticky carrier, such as lanolin or zinc oxide, until it forms a paste that will adhere stubbornly to the skin. This forms an escharotic (caustic) salve that has been successfully employed as a treatment for basal cell cancers on the skin and has even been used for treating internal tumors, especially breast cancer. Another recipe calls for dried, powdered bloodroot mixed with a sticky carrier and zinc chloride, which is itself highly caustic. Although bloodroot salve therapy has apparently been quite effective in many well-publicized cases, it should not be relied upon as a substitute for professional assistance.

Contraindications: Not to be used during pregnancy. For adults only. Bloodroot is an irritant to the gastrointestinal tract—therefore, the rules of low dosage and dilution should be carefully followed. Excessive dosage may also cause nausea and vomiting. Repeated external application to sensitive skin areas may cause pitting or scarring, although it is my experience that using bloodroot to treat tinea and to remove warts normally results in a scar-free resolution. Do not chew the fresh or dried root.

Processing cautions: When grinding dried bloodroot, a filter mask must always be worn. The herb emits an acrid dust that can severely irritate the upper respiratory tract.

Blue Cohosh (*Caulophyllum thalictroides*)
Family: Barberry (*Berberidaceae*)

Parts used: Rhizome and roots (the root) dug during dormancy and used fresh or dried.

Tincture of fresh root: 1:2 (75A:25W)

Tincture of dried root: 1:5 (50A:50W)

Water extracts: Basic tea of the fresh, sliced roots. Basic decoction of the dried root.

Practical uses: Blue cohosh has a profound normalizing effect on the uterus, stemming excessive menstruation or bringing on a delayed menstrual period, as need dictates. The herb will promote regular menstrual discharge, while lessening the severity of cramping. Blue cohosh has traditionally been used during over-term pregnancies and during childbirth, to reduce the incidence of false labor pains, assist in easy delivery, lessen pain in labor, increase the effectiveness of contractions (speed dilation), facilitate delivery of the placenta, and support rapid recovery after birth. See "Contraindications."

Dosage: According to basic recommendations found under "Dosage of tinctures," pages 49–52 and "Dosage of teas and decoctions," pages 70–71. Do not exceed recommended dosage.

Contraindications: Ingestion of blue cohosh signals the pituitary gland to orchestrate increased production of the hormone oxytocin, which stimulates labor, increases the force of contractions, and helps contract the uterine muscle after delivery of the placenta. In prescribing this herb, most modern herbalists suggest that it should not be used during pregnancy, due to the possible risk of miscarriage. A conservative approach is to use this herb only during childbirth, in the instance of slow dilation accompanied by exhaustion. Combine with marshmallow to reduce acridity of the blue cohosh.

Processing cautions: When grinding dried blue cohosh roots, a filter mask should always be worn. The herb emits an acrid dust that can severely irritate the upper respiratory tract.

Blue Flag (*Iris versicolor, I. missouriensis*)
Family: Iris (*Iridaceae*)

Part used: Entire rhizome (the root) dug during growth cycle or dormancy, but preferably not when in full flower. The herb may be used fresh or dried.

Tincture of fresh root: 1:2 (100A)

Tincture of recently dried root: 1:5 (75A:25W)

Practical uses: Blue flag increases bile and pancreatic secretions, thereby aiding in assimilation of fats in the diet and helping dry up oily skin and acne. The herb improves lymphatic function, reduces swollen glands, and assists in the removal of metabolic wastes from the body.

Dosage: This is on the verge of being a low-dose botanical. Typical adult dosage is 5 to 15 drops taken up to 3 times daily, well-diluted in a full cup of water—not for long-term use.

Contraindications: Not to be used during pregnancy or in the presence of overt liver disease. For teenagers and adults only. Do not chew the fresh or dried rhizome; it is quite acrid, and taken thus undiluted will almost certainly irritate the mucous membranes of mouth and throat. Overdose or extreme sensitivity may cause nausea and vomiting.

Processing cautions: When grinding dried blue flag roots, a filter mask must always be worn. The herb emits an acrid dust that can severely irritate the upper respiratory tract.

Boneset (*Eupatorium perfoliatum*)
Family: Aster (*Asteraceae*)

Parts used: Leaf and flowering tops, without the stem, harvested during early flowering stage and used fresh or dried.

Tincture of fresh herb: 1:2 (75A:25W)

Tincture of dried herb: 1:5 (50A:50W)

Water extract: Basic tea or decoction. Cold infusion of the dried herb.

Practical uses: Boneset stimulates the immune response, and is best used during the secondary phases of colds and flu (i.e. swelling of mucous membranes and yellow phlegm.) Using this herb speeds the resolution of infections and supports rapid convalescence. The specific indications are upper respiratory infection—especially if accompanied by aches and pains. This includes: chronic cough, pneumonia, malarial chills, and fevers. Boneset is intensely bitter and gently laxative. Boneset, echinacea, and wild indigo are commonly used in combination to treat influenza.

Dosage: According to basic recommendations found under "Dosage of tinctures," pages 49–52 and "Dosage of teas and decoctions," pages 70–71.

Contraindications: This is a strong herb that should be used only when needed. Excessive dosage will cause purging. The herb is related to gravel root (*Eupatorium purpureum*). The aerial parts of gravel root contain the potentially liver-damaging PAs. Due to conflicting reports, it is not clear whether or not boneset contains PAs. Until this issue can be better elucidated, it is prudent not to use boneset during pregnancy or in the presence of overt liver disease.

Other species: See "Gravel Root."

Brahmi (*Bacopa monnieri*)
Family: Figwort (*Scrophulariaceae*)

Parts used: Aerial portions, including succulent leaves, stems, and flowers if present. The herb is used fresh or dried.

Tincture of fresh herb: 1:2 (50A:50W)

Tincture of dry herb: 1:4 (25A:75W)

Succus of fresh leaves and stems: 1 part alcohol by vol.:3 parts Brahmi juice by vol. (see "Chapter 9, Herbal Succi and Syrups," pages 74–75).

Water extracts: Basic tea of the recently dried leaves and stems.

Direct consumption: The fresh leaf and stem may be plucked from the growing plant and eaten as-is. The plant works at low dosage, is so bitter that one can hardly eat much of it, and grows so fast that a single plant, flourishing in the moist shade in the greenhouse or summer garden, would probably produce a sufficiency for an entire family.

Poultice: To treat cough or bronchitis, make a hot brahmi poultice. Drape a clean, soft cloth over a plate. Steam or briefly boil a double-handful of the brahmi leaves and stems. Place the leafy mass on the cloth, allow it to cool sufficiently so it will not burn the patient, then slide the cloth off the plate onto the bare chest. Cover with plastic, insulate with towels and leave on for at least 20 minutes. This helps break up catarrh and eases breathing. See page 93.

Practical uses: Brahmi enhances mental clarity. Daily use of the plant will improve all aspects of mental function, including rate of learning, retention of information, and problem-solving. Brahmi enhances focus during meditation and helps relieve stress. The plant is used in treatment of mental fatigue, learning disability, attention deficit, addiction, psychosis, autism, epilepsy, neuralgia, and dementia. Combined with ashwagandha, it is good for treating sexual exhaustion. Combined with Saint John's wort, it is good for treating depression. Combined with wood betony, it is good for treating addiction. Brahmi is one of the *rasayana*, a rejuvenating herb that helps one lead a long, fruitful life. It is worth having around!

Dosage: According to basic recommendations found under "Dosage of tinctures," pages 49–52, "Dosage of teas and decoctions," pages 70–71, and "Dosage of succi, page 75." A little goes a long way—start at the lowest listed dosage and work up to moderate dosage over time.

Contraindications: Overdose can cause headache or nausea, which will dissipate once use is discontinued. Do not use concurrently with antidepressants or anti-seizure pharmaceuticals.

Bugle (*Ajuga reptans*)
Family: Mint (*Lamiaceae*)

Parts used: The entire aerial plant, including leaves, stems, and flowers, picked after the morning dew has evaporated, and used fresh or dried.

Tincture of dried herb: 1:5 (50A:40W:10Gly)

Tincture of fresh herb: 1:2 (65A:25W:10Gly)

Water extracts: Basic tea or decoction of the dried herb.

External use: A poultice of fresh bugle leaves, the tea of the dried herb, or tincture of the fresh or dried herb may be used externally as a pain-relieving, anti-inflammatory, and healing embrocation for treating insect stings, ulcerations, and wounds. Use the tea, or dilute the tincture at the rate of 2 droppersful in 1 cup of water (240 ml). Apply to a cloth and hold to the area until relief is achieved. To make a poultice, worry the fresh leaves until juice exudes, then plaster to the affected area.

Oil, salve, or cream: Make infused herbal oil of the fresh herb. This can be used as-is or may be further processed into salve or cream (see "Chapter 10, Basic Formulas for Herbal Oils, Salves, and Creams," page 83, also pages 87–90). Oily preparations of fresh bugle leaves are used to treat wounds or deep bruises.

Practical uses: The tea or tincture have long been held in high repute as a "woundwort," that is an herb which helps heal wounds, whether internal or external. Tenacious coughs, spitting of mucus or blood, external ulcerations, athletic injuries, twisted ankles, tendonitis, and deep bruising may be healed by taking the herb internally and also applying externally.

Dosage: According to basic recommendations found under "Dosage of tinctures," pages 49–52 and "Dosage of teas and decoctions," pages 70–71.

Contraindications: None known. Safe for general use.

Bugleweed (Gipsywort)
(*Lycopus americanus, L. europaeus, L. virginicus*)
Family: Mint (*Lamiaceae*)

Parts used: Fresh or dried leaf and flower, without the stem.

Tincture of fresh herb: 1:2 (75A:25W)

Tincture of dry herb: 1:5 (50A:50W)

Water extracts: Basic tea or decoction.

Practical uses: As a thyroxin antagonist, bugleweed has been successfully utilized for treating hyperthyroidism (overactive thyroid function). The herb is also a valuable heart tonic, used to address arrhythmia, heart disease, and weak heart. Other indications for the use of bugleweed are diarrhea, chronic debilitating cough, insomnia, and hemorrhage of stomach or lungs resulting in expectoration of blood.

Dosage: According to basic recommendations found under "Dosage of tinctures," pages 49–52 and "Dosage of teas and decoctions," pages 70–71.

Contraindications: Not to be used during pregnancy. Clearly inappropriate for use if there is a history of hypothyroidism.

Burdock (*Arctium lappa, A. minus*)
Family: Aster (*Asteraceae*)

Parts used: Root dug during the first growing season and used fresh or dried. Seeds harvested at maturity in the fall of the second growing season and dried.

Tincture of fresh root: 1:2 (75A:25W)

Tincture of dry root (preferred): 1:5 (50A:50W)

Tincture of seed (very strong): 1:4 (75A:25W)
The seeds may be ground up or bruised, soaked overnight in the menstruum, then briefly blended the following day and macerated in the usual manner.

Water extracts: Basic decoction of dried root or seeds.

Practical uses: Fresh burdock root or the various liquid extracts are taken internally as a treatment for staph infections, impetigo, and obstinate ulcerations of the skin or mucous membranes. Often combined with dandelion or yellow dock, burdock is an effective blood purifier used to treat psoriasis, eczema, oily skin, acne, boils, and gout. For treating cancer, burdock is often combined with red clover.

Dosage: According to basic recommendations found under "Dosage of tinctures," pages 49–52 and "Dosage of teas and decoctions," pages 70–71.

Food use: Fresh burdock root is eaten as a medicinal vegetable— boiled, steamed, or used as an ingredient in stir-fry. The raw root is excellent when grated and marinated. Soup is prepared by boiling pieces of the fresh root along with other root vegetables, shiitake, and edible herbs (astragalus, dang-shen, etc.) until all ingredients are thoroughly cooked. The soup is then removed from the heat, the astragalus is fished out, and a tablespoonful or more of miso is stirred in. Served hot, this soup will fortify the system against disease or, if taken by the convalescent, will help to strengthen all body systems and accelerate recovery.

Poultice: The steamed roots are mashed and applied to the affected area as hot as can be tolerated. The fresh leaves may be lightly steamed until flexible and applied hot. This poultice draws out splinters, poisons and suppuration, improves blood flow to injured or infected areas, fights infection, and speeds the healing process.

Contraindications: Burdock root is safe for use as a food. Burdock poultices are also safe for general usage. Burdock decoction and tincture are safe for general use, but it should be understood that, used alone, the herb will sometimes cause expulsion of toxins through the skin, resulting in the formation of pustules. Therefore, burdock is usually combined with a diuretic, such as dandelion, in order to help move toxins out through the urine—not the skin. The intensely bitter seed extract is stronger medicine and should not be used during the first 2 trimesters of pregnancy.

Butterbur (Petasites)
(*Petasites officinalis, P. palmatus*)
Family: Aster (*Asteraceae*)

Parts used: Dormant rhizome used fresh or dried. Stem and leaves picked at maturity and used fresh or dried.

Tincture of fresh rhizome or leaves (preferred): 1:2 (75A:25W)

Tincture of recently dried rhizome or leaves: 1:5 (50A:50W)

Water extracts: Basic tea of the mature, dried leaves or decoction of the dried leaves or rhizomes.

Practical uses: Butterbur is a pain-relieving antispasmodic, used for treating dry, irritated coughs. The pain-relieving aspect is most useful for treating deep-seated afflictions, such as: arthritis, migraine, menstrual cramps, muscle spasms, osteoporosis, and the pain attending various types of cancer.

Dosage: Only as much as is required to do the work—that is, lessen the incidence of coughing or deaden the pain. A good starting dosage is 20 drops of the tincture, 1 cup of tea, or ½ cup of the decoction. Due to the presence of pyrrolizidine alkaloids, the herb should be taken only as needed for acute phase conditions and not on an ongoing basis.

Poultice: The fresh leaves or rhizomes can be bruised or mashed and applied to injuries in order to reduce pain.

Contraindications: Butterbur root and aerial parts contain small quantities of pyrrolizidine alkaloids (PAs) that are potentially liver-toxic substances. Therefore, use of butterbur is contraindicated during pregnancy or nursing, or if there is a history of jaundice or liver disease. The use of petasites for poulticing is safe for anyone.

Other species:[14] There are 15 species of the *Petasites* genus found worldwide. The native uses range widely and the various species contain differing concentrations of the main active compound (petasin), as well as different quantities of PAs. Furthermore, *Petasites* species hybridize and intergrade quite freely. Finally, the concentration of active constituents and PAs may be determined as much by environment, stage of growth, or plant part, as it is by genetics. In the absence of constituent analysis and a careful breeding program, *Petasites* presents a mixed bag at best. There is plenty of room here for further investigation into this beautiful, useful, and fascinating genus.

---

[14]There is confusion between butterbur (*Petasites palmatus*, a plant of the western states) and coltsfoot (*Tussilago farfara*, a plant of the eastern states). This is partially due to the fact that butterbur is sometimes erroneously called "coltsfoot." Butterbur and coltsfoot have similar effects, and although they do not occupy the same native range, they prefer a similar aquatic niche. Their flowering habits are also very similar, since they both flower in the early spring, sometimes prior to the development of leaves. Also, they both contain PAs. Using the Latin names in this case alleviates confusion and miscommunication.

Cactus Grandiflorus (*Selenicereus grandiflorus*)
Family: Cactus (*Cactaceae*)

Parts used: Fresh stem harvested at any time during the growing season—ideally when the plant is in bud and flower. (This usually occurs once per year, during a full moon in the summer.)

Tincture of fresh herb: 1:2 (50A:50W)

Practical uses: Cactus grandiflorus is a heart tonic that is specifically employed for treating poor circulation and cardiac problems arising out of weak nerve force. The herb is an effective treatment for depression caused by drug use, stress, worry, or menopause—especially if these conditions are accompanied by heart malfunction. Cactus is usually combined with other heart tonics, such as hawthorn, garlic, and motherwort.

Dosage: This is a low-dose botanical. Normal adult dosage is 5-15 drops of the tincture taken up to 3 times daily.

Contraindications: Overdose can cause gastric irritation, mental confusion, and may adversely affect the heart muscle.

Pressing: The macerating tincture is highly mucilaginous and may be very slow to press. It is recommended to use 4 layers of cheesecloth instead of heavy pressing cloth, and press in small increments (1 liter at a time) in order to optimize yields.

Calamus (*Acorus calamus; A. americanus*)
Family: Arum (*Araceae*)

Part used: The running rhizome (the root) used fresh or dried. Remove the rootlets from the rhizome; they are medicinally inert.

Tincture of fresh root: 1:2 (100A)

Tincture of dried root: 1:5 (75A:25W)

Acetum of fresh root: 1:2 (100ACV)

Water extract: Basic tea made by stirring 1 teaspoon of the powdered, dried root into 1 cup of hot water.

Direct consumption: Chew a bit of the fresh or dried root.

Practical uses: Calamus is an excellent aromatic bitter for treating indigestion. It is a general stimulant and antispasmodic. Chewing the root is a good treatment for tobacco addiction. It also helps sharpen memory compromised by drug burnout or senility.

Dosage: According to basic recommendations found under "Dosage of tinctures," pages 49–52 and "Dosage of teas and decoctions," pages 70–71. The dosage of the fresh root acetum is 1 tablespoonful (5 ml) taken up to 3 times daily.

Contraindications: The potentially carcinogenic compound known as beta-asarone is present in calamus, with generally higher proportions contained in herb coming from Europe (*Acorus calamus*), as opposed to the North American type (known as *A. americanus* or *A. calamus* var. *americanus*). It is my opinion that beta-asarone is not sufficiently concentrated to pose a threat to those who make occasional use of this herb.

Calendula (*Calendula officinalis*)
Family: Aster (*Asteraceae*)

Parts used: Whole flowers, including the sticky, green calyx, harvested at their peak in the afternoon and used fresh or dried.

Tincture of fresh flowers: 1:2 (100A)

Tincture of dried flowers (preferred): 1:5 (75A:25W)

Water extract: Basic tea. In tea, the flowers are generally combined with other ingredients, such as mullein and marshmallow, for treating hoarseness of voice or upper respiratory infection.

Practical uses: Calendula is most appropriately used externally for its antiseptic and healing properties. The tea or the tincture in water can be swished and swallowed in order to help heal oral lesions, sore throat, or gastric ulcer. For treating traumatic injury, combine calendula with arnica and Saint John's wort.

Dosage: According to basic recommendations found under "Dosage of tinctures," pages 49–52 and "Dosage of teas and decoctions," pages 70–71.

Succus of fresh flowers: 1 part alcohol by vol.:3 parts calendula flower juice by vol. (see "Chapter 9, Herbal Succi and Syrups," pages 73–75). Calendula succus is a low-alcohol extract that delivers the same antiseptic activity as calendula tincture, but is kinder to open wounds, abrasions, surgical cuts, and sutures. Use of this succus is especially indicated as an antiseptic and healing wash following gynecological procedures or surgery.

External use: Calendula is most often used externally as an antiseptic, anti-inflammatory, and healing wash or compress for insect stings, ulcerations, varicose ulcers, wounds, and old burns. Use the tea, the succus, or dilute the tincture at the rate of 2 droppersful in 1 cup of water (240 ml). Full strength, calendula tincture or succus may be briskly rubbed on the legs or torso to help shrink and heal spider veins and varicose veins.

Oil, salve, or cream: Make infused herbal oil of the dried flowers. This can be used as-is or may be further processed into salve or cream (see "Chapter 10, Basic Formulas for Herbal Oils, Salves, and Creams," pages 85–90). These products are for external use as an anti-inflammatory and antiseptic application for treating cuts, old burns, abrasions, sunburn, chapped skin, diaper rash, or as a general cosmetic.

Food use: The flower petals (actually the ray flowers) make a harmless and colorful decoration for summer salads.

Contraindications: Safe for external use. Safe for internal use at stated dosage. Overdose of calendula taken internally may cause stomach upset, nausea, or emesis.

Cultivars: Calendula has been selected over time to produce various strains, some of which are rich in medicinally active flavonoids and resins, while others are medicinally deficient. The purely horticultural strains such as "Pacific Beauty" are very pretty, but the resin content may be extremely low. Strains selected for high resin content are recommended. If the fresh flowers leave a thick, dark, sticky exudate on your fingers when you pick a few hundred flowers or so, this is ample proof that you are working with a strain of high resin content. Both orange and yellow, double and single flowers can be excellent.

Cascara Sagrada (Chittam) (*Rhamnus purshiana*)
Family: Buckthorn (*Rhamnaceae*)

Part used: Bark, sliced and peeled from the wood in the spring, dried, then aged for at least 1 year before use. Aging is best accomplished by keeping the bark pieces in breathable sacks (washed burlap) in an airy, dry, and dark location.

Tincture of dried, aged bark: 1:5 (75A:25W)

Water extract: Basic cold infusion, started in the morning for use just before bed. Basic decoction.

Syrup: Combine 1 part of the strong decoction with 2 parts of honey. Follow procedure found in "Chapter 9, Herbal Succi and Syrups."

Practical uses: Cascara sagrada is a remarkable laxative acting on the large intestine and is generally astringent and tonifying to the gastrointestinal tract. The herb is useful for softening the stools in the case of anal fissure, hemorrhoids, or postoperative situations. Effects are not usually apparent until at least 6 hours after the first dosage. Taking the extract before bed usually results in a bowel movement immediately upon waking in the morning. Repeated dosage in the first 6 hours may cause an unintended overdose. Taking the herb in combination with a carminative, such as: anise, fennel, calamus, or lemon balm will reduce cramping. In any case, a "moving" experience.

Dosage of the tincture: 1 to 2 droppersful (30 to 60 drops) taken just before bed.

Dosage of the cold infusion: ½ to 1 cup (120 to 240 ml) before bed.

Dosage of the syrup: 2 tablespoonsful (30 ml) before bed. When using this herb, it is best to begin with low dosage and adjust on future occasions according to the degree of response.

Contraindications: Not to be taken during pregnancy or nursing; the effects will go through the milk to the child. Use of the green (uncured) bark will result in intense intestinal cramping. Overdose of the cured bark may prove similarly uncomfortable. Cascara sagrada should not be taken in the case of diarrhea, intestinal cramping, or obstruction. Dependency can develop. Frequent and prolonged use may result in loss of water and potassium salts, which can potentiate the effects of heart medicines containing cardiac glycosides.

Processing cautions: Gloves should be worn when handling quantities of the green, undried bark. The side effects resulting from getting the green juices on the hands are the same as the practical uses, but more violent, and less convenient.

Other species: Buckthorn *(Rhamnus catharticus)* cured bark is, for all practical purposes, interchangeable with cascara sagrada.

Catnip (*Nepeta cataria*)
Family: Mint (*Lamiaceae*)

Parts used: Leaf and flower harvested in early flowering stage, without the stem, used fresh or dried.

Tincture of fresh herb: 1:2 (75A:25W)

Tincture of dried herb: 1:5 (50A:50W)

Water extract: Basic tea of fresh or dried herb.

Practical uses: Catnip is a gentle antispasmodic for relieving indigestion and gas. The herb is a mild and specific remedy for infant colic. The warm tea is often effective in bringing on a delayed menstrual period. It is also used as a sedative for treating sleeplessness, for dispelling headache, and sweating out fever. Of course, it is a favorite of cats, some of which develop an almost unnatural affection for it. The bruised, fresh herb may be given to cats, to make them happy or to silence nighttime yowling.

Dosage: According to basic recommendations found under "Dosage of tinctures," pages 49–52 and "Dosage of teas and decoctions," pages 70–71.

Contraindications: Not to be used during pregnancy.

Other species: There are about 250 species of perennial herbs in the *Nepeta* genus. Many of these, including Syrian catnip (*N. curvifolia*) and catmint (*N. faassenii*) are quite aromatic and may be used as tea herbs for good taste and digestive effects.

Celandine (*Chelidonium majus*)
Family: Poppy (*Papaveraceae*)

Parts used: Whole plant, including root, leaf, stem, and flowers, harvested in the spring during full flower and used fresh or dried.

Acetous tincture of fresh plant: 1:2 (75A:25ACV)

Acetous tincture of dried plant: 1:5 (50A:50ACV); see page 56.

Water extract: Basic tea. Use only 1 teaspoonful (~1 g) of the dried herb per cup (240 ml) of water, taken 2 or 3 times daily. Do not exceed recommended dose. Not for extended use.

Practical uses: Celandine is an alterative, an herb that helps to re-establish healthy functions of the immune system, especially in the case of organ stasis and wasting diseases. The herb is stimulating to the liver and antispasmodic to the gastrointestinal tract. Celandine is also prophylactic against cancer and is sometimes used to treat cancer—helps free up and disperse toxins.

Dosage: This is a low-dose botanical. Normal adult dosage is 5 to 15 drops of the acetous tincture taken 2 or 3 times daily, well-diluted in at least 1 cup of water.

External: As an alterative hand or foot soak, make 1 quart of strong tea, pour this into a basin of hot water, and soak for 20 minutes. This is of assistance in treating malaise of the entire body system—not just the hands or feet. The advantage of this mode of administration is its gentle, yet powerful, alterative effect. As a treatment for warts, the orange latex that exudes from broken pieces of the fresh plant or root may be carefully applied directly to the wart twice daily until it dries up and falls off. Not effective for treating plantar warts. The acetous tincture is generally too weak to work against warts, but full-strength juice may prove effective against abnormal skin growths.

Contraindications: Not to be used during pregnancy. For adults only. Excessive dosage may cause gastrointestinal upset or nausea. Do not chew on the fresh plant, no matter how inviting it looks. The fresh juices are extremely acrid and, applied thus undiluted, will irritate the mucous membranes of mouth and throat. To protect mucosa, combine with marshmallow.

Chameleon Plant (Yu-xing-cao, Fishwort)
(*Houttuynia cordata*)
Family: Lizard's Tail (*Saururaceae*)

Parts used: Leaves and rhizomes collected prior to flowering, and used fresh. Dried leaves.

Tincture of whole fresh plant: 1:2 (50A:50W)

Glycerite of whole fresh plant: 1:2 (100 Gly)

Water extracts: Decoction of the dried leaves is useful in treating dysentery. The leaves should be soaked overnight and very briefly simmered (less than 5 minutes) the next morning. Antibacterial compounds in this plant are heat-labile and prolonged heating will reduce efficacy.

Practical uses: This is one of the Chinese herbs that clears heat, resolves toxicity, and reduces swelling. Lung infections, especially if associated with profuse discharge, yield to the tincture or direct consumption. Purulent sores may be treated by poulticing with the fresh, pulverized herb while taking the tincture or glycerite internally. The herb is a broad-spectrum antiviral and antibacterial, has the ability to disperse toxins, and may be found useful in treating urinary tract infections, *Mycoplasma* (very tiny gram-positive bacteria responsible for a plethora of health-woes and often associated with lyme disease), herpes simplex, dengue virus, avian flu, zika virus, West Nile virus and candidiasis.

Dosage: According to basic recommendations found under "Dosage of tinctures," pages 49–52 and "Dosage of teas and decoctions," pages 70–71.

Food use: The fresh leaves have a lemony taste with deep, fishy undertones and are consumed in salads, in fresh spring rolls, and with noodles. The rhizomes are long, thin, white, and crisp, delicious when chopped and added to soups or fish curry. I saw whole tables loaded with the fresh, bundled rhizomes when visiting Kunming vegetable market in Yunnan Province, China—the herb is quite popular there. Noticing my interest, a kind vendor gifted me with a small bundle, which I wrapped in moist paper, keeping it alive until I was able to plant it in my home garden. I was lucky—he had provided me with the species plant.

Contraindications: Subcutaneous injection of the herb has caused serious side effects. The herb should not be injected, rather taken orally, fresh or tinctured, in which case there are no known side effects.

Other species: There are many horticultural selections of different colors and variegations. However, the medicine should be made from the species plant, with its homogenously green leaves.

Chamomile, German
(*Matricaria recutita* syn. *Matricaria chamomilla*)
Family: Aster (*Asteraceae*)

Part used: The entire flowers picked at peak development, in the morning after the dew has barely evaporated, and used fresh or dried.

Tincture of fresh flowers: 1:2 (75A:25W)

Tincture of dried flowers: 1:5 (50A:50W)

Glycerite of fresh flowers: 1:2 (100Gly); see page 61.

Water extract: Basic tea of fresh or (preferably) dried flowers.

Practical uses: Chamomile makes a delightfully fragrant tea, calming to the stomach. Taken after the evening meal to improve digestion, the herb will also help calm the nervousness leftover from a busy and challenging day and promote deep sleep. Chamomile is antispasmodic to the intestinal tract and helps heal gastric and duodenal ulcers. In this application, the herb combines well with licorice.

Dosage: According to basic recommendations found under "Dosage of tinctures," pages 49–52 and "Dosage of teas and decoctions," pages 70–71.

External: A quart of strong tea added to a basin of hot Epsom salt water makes an excellent antibacterial soak or compress for treating localized infections. Alternately, use 1 teaspoonful (5 ml) of the tincture in the Epsom salt water. To soothe sore eyes, soak chamomile tea bags in a small amount of hot water (just enough to thoroughly soften the herb), then allow the tea bags to cool. Lie down, relax, and place them on your closed eyes.   For enlivening blonde hair, make 1 quart of strong tea and use, at luke-warm temperature, after shampooing, as a rinse. This improves the color and texture of the hair, imparting a delightful fragrance.

Contraindications: Some individuals will experience headache as a side effect of taking chamomile. Do not take if there is a known allergy to the *Asteraceae.* Avoid direct contact with pure, undiluted essential oil of chamomile—especially on sensitive skin, mucous membranes, and in eyes.

Other species: Although classed in a different genus, Roman chamomile (*Chamaemelum nobile*) is closely allied to German chamomile (*Matricaria recutita*) and the two are medicinally interchangeable. However, German chamomile smells and tastes better and is, therefore, generally preferred. Pineapple weed or "dog fennel" (variously classified as *Matricaria discoidea*, *Chamomilla sauveolens*, or *Matricaria matricarioides*) looks similar to these choice chamomiles, but smells quite obnoxious. Pineapple weed is a poor substitute at best, is likely to produce side effects and is not recommended.   In the case of the chamomiles, knowing the Latin is of little help in communicating about the plant. The taxonomists have not been able to make up their minds about this one, and the plant has more Latin names than it needs. The common names Roman chamomile or German chamomile definitely present a clearer picture to a wider audience than . . . now what is the current binomial?

Chaste Tree (*Vitex agnus-castus*)
Family: Vervain (*Verbenaceae*)

Part used: The berries (also known as the fruits or seeds) har-vested in the autumn at full maturity and dried.

Tincture of dried berries: 1:4 (75A:25W)
The berries must be crushed or milled to a coarse powder before adding the menstruum, then macerated in the usual manner.

Water extract: Basic tea of crushed berries.

Direct consumption: The berries can be taken singly, held in the mouth, and slowly crunched and consumed, one after another, resulting in the desired effects. The dosage is approximately ½ level teaspoon (~1 g) over the course of a day.

Practical uses: The herb has a general hormone-balancing effect, and is commonly used for treating menstrual disorders, premenstrual syndrome (PMS), infertility, endometriosis, and as a galactagogue for increasing milk production. It can also be helpful in reducing the sex drive of over amorous men.

Dosage: According to basic recommendations found under "Dosage of tinctures," pages 49–52 and "Dosage of teas and decoctions," pages 70–71.

Contraindications: The herb is meant to ease menstrual discomfort. If taking chaste berries seems to be *increasing* the symptoms, then discontinue use. Not to be taken during pregnancy or in combination with birth control pills.

Other species: *Vitex* is a genus of about 270 species of shrubs and trees. Although *V. agnus-castus* is official, the berries of nirgundi (*V. negundo*) and the simpleleaf chaste tree (*V. trifolia*) demonstrate similar medicinal activity.

Chickweed (*Stellaria media*)
Family: Pink (*Caryophyllaceae*)

Parts used: Entire herb, including leaf, stem, and flowers, harvested in early flowering stage in the early spring or fall and used fresh or dried. The dried herb makes a better extract, but only if it is recent, bright green, and possessed of the clean, new-mown hay aroma characteristic of quality chickweed.

Tincture of fresh herb: 1:2 (50A:50W)

Tincture of dried herb: 1:5 (25A:75W)

Succus of fresh plant: 1 part alcohol by volume: 3 parts plant juice by volume (see "Chapter 9, Herbal Succi and Syrups").

Water extracts: Basic tea made of fresh or dried herb.

Direct consumption: Chew the fresh leaves and stems in the early spring, when you find them unaccountably covering that entire raised bed you made in the spring of the previous year and had considered to be pretty much weed-free—a consolation prize.

Practical uses: Chickweed is a nourishing tonic for improving overall energy levels. The saponins help scrub toxins from the bloodstream and gastrointestinal system. Many people will experience a mild laxative effect from eating fresh chickweed. The herb has an alkalinizing effect on the blood and is used to treat hyperacidity of diet (generally caused by insufficient intake of fresh greens and grains). The herb helps speed fat metabolism and can be a useful tool in weight reduction programs. The fresh herb is also an excellent hen feed, increasing egg size, overall production, and improving the nutritional value of the eggs.

Dosage: According to basic recommendations found under "Dosage of tinctures," pages 49–52 and "Dosage of teas and decoctions," pages 70–71.

Food use: The fresh herb is delicious in salads, delivering its nutritional and medicinal effects, regardless of admixture with lettuce and other salad ingredients.

Poultice: The mashed or slightly masticated leaves of chickweed make an excellent cooling and healing poultice for treating wounds that will not heal, insect stings, sore eyes, oily skin and acne, or eczema.

Oil, salve, or cream: Make infused herbal oil of the entire dried plant. This can be used as-is or as an ingredient for making salve or cream, according to the procedure found in "Chapter 10, Basic Formulas for Herbal Oils, Salves, and Creams." These products are for external use as an anti-inflammatory treatment for arthritic or rheumatic joints and for helping heal skin rashes or eczema.

Contraindications: None known. Safe for general use. Consuming large amounts of fresh chickweed may cause looseness of stools, which is consistent with the "spring cleanse."

Other species: Stellaria is a cosmopolitan genus that is represented by up to 120 species worldwide, many of them used as tonics by local barefoot doctors. This is an ethnobotanical proving for cross-cultural use of a healing herb. For example, Yunnan chickweed (qian-zhen-wan-xian-cao) (*Stellaria yunnanensis*) is a perennial endemic to Yunnan in China, where the tubers are cooked in soup, being both nutritive and tonic. I once encountered giant African chickweed (*Stellaria mannii*) growing wayside on Pemba Island in Zanzibar. Tasting a leaf, I was immediately reminded of our own temperate species, the slightly soapy sensation at the back of the throat, which is indicative of the presence of saponins. Locals use the herb for food, fodder, and as a rejuvenative tonic.

Cilantro (Coriander)
(*Coriandrum sativum*)
Family: Carrot (*Apiaceae*)

Parts used: Fresh leaves, stems, and green seeds are known as "cilantro" and are used in the culinary arts and for making the tincture. The mature seeds are a schizocarp that splits into two viable hemispheres. The seed is known as "coriander," also used in cooking.

Tincture of fresh cilantro: 1:2 (75A:25W)

Succus of fresh plant: 1 part alcohol by volume:3 parts plant juice by volume (see "Chapter 9, Herbal Succi and Syrups," pages 73–5).

Direct consumption: Chop the fresh leaves and add to your food. Coriander seeds may be ground up and added to foods during the cooking process or as a sprinkle on ready foods.

Practical uses: Most people find cilantro and coriander to be tasty condiments, used in flavoring bean dishes and generally sharpening the appetite. The herb promotes the flow of bile. Consuming fresh cilantro (in food or as a tincture) helps mobilize heavy metals including mercury, cadmium, lead, and aluminum from bones, teeth, central nervous system, and other body tissues. To avoid retoxification from heavy metals that are freed to the bodily tissues, blood, or lymph, combine cilantro tincture with dandelion or red clover tincture (50:50), which helps dispel these toxins through the urine. Alternatively, put the cilantro tincture in water along with 1 teaspoonful of bentonite clay. Stir and drink. This helps chelate heavy metals and moves them out through the bowel. To treat headache, put 20 drops of cilantro tincture in a cup of hot water and slowly sip. Combine cilantro tincture with spilanthes tincture (50:50) in a glass of water and use as an oral swish, post-brushing, to freshen breath, tonify oral mucosa, and help dispel heavy metals from fillings.

Dosage: According to basic recommendations found under "Dosage of tinctures," pages 49–52 and "Dosage of teas and decoctions," pages 70–71. If using the fresh herb tincture or the fresh herb succus, double the dose.

Contraindications: None known. Safe for general use. Some people are genetically predisposed to detest the smell and taste of cilantro. If the herb offend thee, do not use it!

Cleavers (*Galium aparine*)
Family: Madder (*Rubiaceae*)

Parts used: The entire aerial plant, including leaves and stems, harvested in the spring in the early flowering stage and used fresh or dried. The fresh herb has a water content exceeding 90% and can be difficult to dry without spoilage. Protect your cleavers from bruising during harvest (do not crush), spread thinly on the drying screens, turn frequently, and provide good air flow and gentle heat. Under these conditions, the herb will dry in 2 days time.

Tincture of fresh herb: 1:2 (100A)

Tincture of dried herb: 1:5 (50A:50W)

Succus of fresh plant: 1 part alcohol by volume:3 parts plant juice by volume (see "Chapter 9, Herbal Succi and Syrups," pages 73–5). The fresh herb succus is really the best way to take the herb.

Water extracts: Boiling destroys the medicinal virtues of cleavers, so make the basic tea of the dried herb with warm (not hot) water or make a cold infusion of the dried herb.

Practical uses: Cleavers is rich in plant chlorophyll and is one of the premier spring tonics, promoting lymphatic circulation and purifying the blood. The herb is used for treating urinary tract infection and its main symptoms—painful or difficult urination; also used for treating urinary stone, kidney inflammation, and prostatitis. Cleavers is a strong diuretic and also cools and shrinks inflamed tissues of the urinary tract. The herb helps rid the body of metabolic waste, and is useful in treating any illness attended by swollen glands, including tonsillitis and earache. Used internally and applied externally as a wash, the tea, succus, or diluted tincture may be of service in treating poison oak and ivy, sunburn, psoriasis, and other skin eruptions.

Dosage: According to basic recommendations found under "Dosage of tinctures," pages 49–52 and "Dosage of teas and decoctions," pages 70–71. If using the fresh herb tincture or the fresh herb succus, double the dose.

Poultice: It is easy to thoroughly mash the leaves and stems of cleavers, making an excellent cooling and healing poultice for treating poison oak and ivy, open sores, blisters, and burns.

Oil, salve, or cream: Make infused herbal oil of the dried aerial parts of the plant. This can be used as-is or as an ingredient for making salve or cream, according to the procedure found in "Chapter 10, Basic Formulas for Herbal Oils, Salves, and Creams." Cleavers cream promotes a clear complexion. Used in the form of an oil or salve, cleavers may help reduce swollen glands, remove nodular growths on the skin, and shrink tumors—both benign and cancerous.

Contraindications: None known. Safe for general use

Clover, Red (*Trifolium pratense*)
Family: Legume (*Fabaceae*)

Parts used: Young blossoms and leaves used fresh or dried.

Tincture of fresh herb: 1:2 (75A:25W)

Tincture of dried herb: 1:5 (50A:50W)

Water extract: Basic tea of the fresh or dried herb.

Practical uses: Red clover is a blood-thinning alterative that helps the body efficiently remove metabolic waste products and

151

prohibits the attachment and metastasis of abnormal cells. This is, therefore, one of the best single supplements for prevention and treatment of cancer. The herb helps maintain normal estrogen levels during menopause for maintenance of healthy bones, skin, and arteries, helps normalize blood pressure and cholesterol levels, and promotes youthfulness.

Dosage: According to basic recommendations found under "Dosage of tinctures," pages 49–52 and "Dosage of teas and decoctions," pages 70–71.

Poultice: The fresh herb is chopped, combined with a little water, and mashed or blended, then applied directly to abnormal lesions.

Contraindications: Not to be used during pregnancy. Cancer is a serious illness that must be attended by a qualified health professional. Do not take red clover along with melilot (*Melilotus officinalis*) or with the pharmaceutical anticoagulant coumadin or warfarin. The blood-thinning effects may be noticeable as an increased tendency to bleed from cuts and a longer time required for coagulation.

Other species: The edibility and medicinal applications of the 300 species that make up the *Trifolium* genus is an inadequately studied subject begging for further research. Traditionally, most of the clovers have been cultivated as cover crops, forage crops, and for making hay. Aztec clover (*T. amabile*) and several other indigenous American clovers including *T. ciliatum, T. gracilentum,* and *T. tridentatum* were used historically as foodstuffs by Native Americans. Besides red clover (*T. pratense*), which is considered official, the main species employed for making tea are Alsike clover (*T. hybridum*), crimson clover (*T. incarnatum*), and white clover (*T. repens*). Although the apparent safety of the tea of these clovers has been established, their potential utility as blood-thinning alteratives is not adequately confirmed. See "Melilot."

Comfrey (*Symphytum officinale*)
Family: Borage (*Boraginaceae*)

Parts used: Root dug from fall through spring. Leaf harvested when fully formed, but prior to flowering. The cell-proliferating molecule alantoin tends to be present at highest levels when and where the plant is growing fastest. If the plant is dormant, the allantoin resides in the root. Comfrey may be used fresh or dried. After flowering, the plants are cut back, mulched with their own leaves, and allowed to grow back through this cushy mulch. Comfrey builds soil.

Tincture of fresh root: 1:2 (50A:50W)
The alcohol content of this tincture is kept to a minimum, since alcohol causes the healing mucilage to precipitate in globs. Due to the thick viscosity of comfrey tincture, it is important to press slowly and at low pressure. Filter through cheesecloth.

Water extract: Cold infusion of dried leaf.

Practical uses: Comfrey speeds healing of cuts, ulcerations, bruises, broken bones, pulled muscles and ligaments, and sprains.

Dosage: According to basic recommendations found under "Dosage of tinctures," pages 49–52 and "Dosage of teas and decoctions," pages 70–71. See "Contraindications."

Oil, salve, or cream: Make infused herbal oil of the dried root or dried leaves. This oil can be used as-is or as an ingredient for making salve or cream, (see "Chapter 10, Basic Formulas for Herbal Oils, Salves, and Creams," pages 83–90).

Poultice: The poultice of dried root or fresh plant is described in detail in "Chapter 11, Poultices, Compresses, and Soaks," page 97. The poultice speeds healing of traumatic injury and relieves pain.

Contraindications: Do not use when pregnant or nursing. Ingesting large quantities of comfrey during pregnancy or using large comfrey poultices daily during pregnancy has been associated with the risk of infant hepatic veno-occlusive disease. Comfrey contains pyrrolizidine alkaloids (PAs), which are a potential liver toxin. The PAs are of higher concentration in the root than in the leaves. Taken internally, a 3-week course of comfrey root extract or comfrey leaf tea is considered harmless to the liver of a healthy, nonpregnant person. Do not take for longer than 3 weeks. For nonpregnant individuals, there is little danger of absorption of toxic levels of PAs through the skin from comfrey salves, creams, and poultices. Do not use this herb externally on new puncture wounds or deep cuts, due to the likelihood that the outer skin layers will be stimulated to close up and heal prior to the draining and regeneration of deeper tissues. Instead, first use Epsom salt soaks containing calendula or chamomile tincture. Once the swelling and pain have subsided and the wound is clean and healing normally, comfrey may be safely and effectively applied to speed the process.

Other species: The origional land-race of Russian comfrey (*Symphytum asperum*), and hybridized types coming from Eastern Europe (e.g. *S. x uplandicum*) are actually higher than *S. officinale* in echimidine, one of the most toxic of the PAs found in comfrey.

Cramp Bark (*Viburnum opulis, V. trilobum*)
Family: Honeysuckle (*Caprifoliaceae*)

Parts used: Stem bark or root bark of the bush, harvested in the spring when the sap is up, the outer and inner bark whittled off the wood into quills. The bark is then dried and ground up before use. When wetted with water, covered in a jar and left overnight, good cramp bark herb will smell like valerian, due to the presence of valerenic acid, which is one of the antispasmodic constituents of this benign and useful herb.

Tincture of dried bark: 1:5 (50A:50W)

Water extract: Basic decoction.

Practical uses: The tincture or decoction treats premenstrual syndrome, dysmenorrhea, painful uterine cramps, or cramps of other smooth muscles including intestines and rectum. The tincture is prescribed by midwives to treat pregnant women suffering from symptoms of miscarriage, including spotting or cramps. The tincture may be prescribed as a prophylactic to those with a history of miscarriage.

Dosage: According to basic recommendations found under "Dosage of tinctures," pages 49–52 and "Dosage of teas and decoctions," pages 70–71.

Contraindications: None known. Safe for general use.

Other species: Black haw (*Viburnum prunifolium*) root bark is used interchangeably with cramp bark. *Viburnum opulus* is the European species, and *V. trilobum* is the North American species. They are used interchangeably in herbal medicine.

Culver's Root
(*Veronicastrum virginicum* syn. *Leptandra virginica*)
Family: Figwort (*Scrophulariaceae*)

Parts used: The rhizome and roots (the root) dug during dormancy, dried, and aged for at least 6 months. Aging is best accomplished by keeping the bark pieces in breathable sacks (washed burlap) in an airy, dry, and dark location.

Tincture of dried, aged root: 1:5 (50A:50W)

Water extract: Basic decoction.

Syrup: Combine 1 part of the strong decoction with 2 parts of honey. Follow procedure found in "Chapter 9, Herbal Succi and Syrups," pages 76–80.

Practical uses: Culver's root is a digestive tonic, improving function of the liver, gall bladder, bile ducts, and intestinal tract. The herb is used specifically for treating gallstones, constipation, gastroenteritis, and chronic indigestion. Low dosage is useful for tonifying the gastrointestinal tract, while higher dosage will prove laxative.

Dosage: Beginning adult dosage of the tincture is 10 to 30 drops, 3 times per day. The beginning dosage of the decoction is ½ cup taken twice daily. The beginning dosage of the syrup is 2 tablespoonsful taken twice daily.

Contraindications: Do not use during pregnancy. Use of the green (undried) root will cause drastic purging.

Curry Leaf Tree (*Murraya koenigii*)
Family: Citrus (*Rutaceae*)

Parts used: Young leaves, used fresh or recently dried. The young leaves (harvested from newer branches) contain a higher concentration of essential oils and oleo-gum-resins than the older leaves, which tend to be quite leathery and inodorous. The fresh leaves are generally preferred to the dried leaves. When refrigerated, the leaves are best left on the stem, to help maintain their potency, but even at that, they don't last long. For best results, grow your own! The bark of the tree and the root are also used in Ayurvedic medicine. They should be peeled or carved from renewable portions of the tree, shade dried and ground to a powder before use.

Tincture of fresh leaves: 1:2 (75A:25W). Remove the leaves from the stems, weigh and place in blender, measure and add the menstruum, blend, then macerate and press in the usual manner.

Water extracts: Basic tea of fresh or dried herb. The tea will benefit from long brewing, and may be put on to steep in the morning and strained and sipped throughout the day. This is a good treatment for weak stomach, lack of appetite, or nausea. The fresh leaves may also be briefly pan-fried before making the tea. This improves speed of extraction, and is the recommended method of preparation for treating morning sickness during pregnancy.

Succus of fresh plant: 1 part alcohol by volume:3 parts plant juice by volume (see "Chapter 9, Herbal Succi and Syrups," pages 73–5). The dosage is 1 teaspoonful of the plain juice or succus, mixed in 1 cup (240 ml) of cow's milk or coconut milk with lime, and taken 2 or 3 times daily, to treat nausea or dysentery.

Direct consumption: Eat 10 leaves in the morning to freshen breath, cleanse the teeth, improve digestion, discourage diabetes, lose weight, increase vital force, and promote longevity.

Culinary use: The spicily aromatic, pinnate leaves of this tropical shrub to small tree are widely employed in the cuisine of Southern India and Sri Lanka, where it is known as *kaddi patta*. The leaves (without the stem) are chopped and stir-fried briefly in oil before the addition of onions, and impart their delightful, citrusy aroma and taste to curries, soups, and other dishes. Using curry leaf in cooking enhances flavor and is kind to the stomach.

Practical uses: Fresh leaves, fresh leaf juice, tincture, or succus may be taken at recommended dosage for treatment of: upset stomach, nausea, constipation, diarrhea, dysentery, hepatitis, anemia, diabetes, heart disease and high cholesterol. The herb also helps protect from radiation damage during chemotherapy, proves antioxidant against systemic free radicals, helps darken the hair, and strengthens the teeth. The dried bark or root bark may be ground to a powder and mixed in water to make a drink to treat vomiting and stomach upset. The dosage is 1 teaspoonful of powder to 1 cup (240 ml) of water. During *homas* and *pujas*, curry leaf may be used as a substitute for holy basil (*Ocimum sanctum*), when the tulsi is not available.

Dosage: According to basic recommendations found under "Dosage of tinctures," pages 49–52 and "Dosage of teas and decoctions," pages 70–71.

Contraindications: None known.

Other species: Murraya is a genus of at least 9 citrusy species, generally employed for their food, medicine, and landscaping appeal. Orange jessamine (*Murraya paniculata*), is an elegant shrub to small tree that is native to China and the Himalayas. Leaves of this tree are used much like curry leaf, as a tonic and stomachic. We once grew this citrus relative as a potted plant in our greenhouse, and it was quite handsome, with shiny, pinnate leaves, studded in season with clusters of waxy, white flowers emitting glorious perfume. I cannot remember when we lost the tree (probably during an icy winter while we were away), but in my mind's nose, the scent still lingers . . .

Dandelion, Common (*Taraxacum officinale*)
Family: Aster (*Asteraceae*)

Parts used: Root or entire plant with root dug in early flowering stage and used fresh or dried.

Tincture of fresh root or fresh flowering plant with root: 1:2 (75A:25W)

Tincture of dried root: 1:5 (50A:50W)

Succus: 1 part alcohol by volume:3 parts expressed juice of ground, fresh flowering plant with root (see pages 74–75).

Water extracts: Basic tea of fresh flowering plant or dried leaves. Decoction of fresh or dried root.

Practical uses: Dandelion is a wild weed that grows well in the domestic garden. It is a classic spring tonic. The herb is somewhat laxative, markedly diuretic, and improves the function of the liver, promoting secretion of bile. As such, dandelion is an excellent blood-cleanser, helping rid the system of accumulated toxins and improving bad skin. The herb is commonly combined with burdock in treatment of staph. Dandelion also combines well with lomatium, and indeed is a necessary part of lomatium therapy. The fresh flowers are traditionally used to make dandelion wine or dandelion beer, beverages that retain the blood-cleansing activity of the herb.

Dosage: According to basic recommendations found under "Dosage of tinctures," pages 49–52 and "Dosage of teas and decoctions," pages 70–71.

Food use: The fresh buds and flowers are a cleansing, yet fortifying, trailside snack. Obviously, care needs to be taken when harvesting flowers in urban areas, due to the high incidence of chemical applications and doggy applications. It is my personal opinion that in cities, the grass should be discouraged in preference to the dandelions, not the other way around. The fresh greens are an excellent salad ingredient.

Contraindications: In the case of gallbladder inflammation or gallstones, dandelion should be used only under the advice and care of a qualified health professional.

Other species: There are over 50 species in the *Taraxacum* genus, all taprooted biennials or perennials that contain milky latex. *T. hybernum* has been cultivated for production of rubber. Red-seeded dandelion (*T. erythrospermum*) and Chinese dandelion (pu-gong-ying) (*T. mongolicum*) are used interchangeably with common dandelion for their diuretic and alterative effects. At least four distinct cultivars have been produced from common dandelion. One of these, French dandelion, bears large, broad leaves arranged in a clump instead of a simple rosette. This plant will generally produce more leaf mass per plant than common dandelion, which is of advantage for salad making.

Dan-shen (Chinese Red Sage) (*Salvia miltiorrhiza*) Family: Mint (*Lamiaceae*)

Parts used: The root of 6 month or older plants, dug during dormancy (late fall to early spring) and dried. Shake root mass free of dirt and wash gently so as to preserve the red pigment that resides on the outer surface. This pigment is indicative of the presence of the lipophilic diterpene quinone molecules known as tanshinones, the main active constituents of dan-shen. Use only the taproots, not the hair roots or crown of the plant. Briefly air dry, then slice the roots obliquely and place on screens in the shade, and dry until the pieces snap. The decoction may be made from these pieces without further grinding, but to make the tincture, the root must first be ground to a coarse powder.

Tincture: 1:4 (75A:25W) Tincturing is a cold process and high alcohol content is required in order to extract the tanshinone molecules. The tincture is the best dosage form for daily use by men as a heart tonic and prophylactic against heart attack and stroke.

Water extracts: Standard decoction. The decoction is a hot process, which increases the solubility of the active constituents in water. The decoction is the best dosage form for treating menstrual woes and for short-term usage when a high dose is desired.

Practical uses: Dan-shen is one of the main herbs of traditional Chinese medicine that regulates the blood. This herb decreases blood viscosity, dissolves and dispels clots, dilates the coronary arteries, slows and strengthens the heart beat, helps reduce blood cholesterol, fights atherosclerosis, and improves circulation to the tiny capillaries that surround the vital organs, including especially the heart. Lack of circulation to the heart muscle is the main cause of stroke and heart attack, where blood clots form in any of the three coronary arteries and may break free and circulate, eventually blocking blood flow to the brain, lungs, or heart. Cold extremities, chest pain (angina), painful menses, and postpartum abdominal pain, fibroid cysts and breast abscess may also yield to therapy with dan-shen. See "Contraindications."

Dosage: According to basic recommendations found under "Dosage of tinctures," pages 49–52. The decoction is made of 30 grams of root and yields 4 cups (see page 69). The recommended dosage is 15 grams per day, so drinking 1 cup of decoction in the morning, and 1 cup at night achieves the correct daily dosage. The remaining decoction may be refrigerated and utilized the next day. See "Contraindications."

Contraindications: Not to be used during pregnancy. May potentiate the effects of blood thinners and should not be used by those taking coumarin, warfarin, aspirin, or nonsteroidal anti-inflammatories (NSAIDS). Dan-shen is proestrogenic, and increased estrogen can be a contributing factor to breast cancer. Therefore, women taking this herb to relieve menstrual pain or post-partum pain should use only as needed, not on a long-term basis. Women should not take this herb for longer than 1 month running, and then discontinue for another month before taking it again. Men, on the other hand, especially when at-risk, can take dan-shen tincture on a daily basis as a prophylactic against atherosclerosis, heart disease, heart attack, and stroke.

Other species: Other members of the family *Lamiaceae* also contain the active constituent tanshinone, most notably California chia (*Salvia columbariae*). This little desert dweller is also known by the native name "ilipesh," which translates "to wake the dead," in reference to its traditional use for resuscitating victims of stroke.

I have a strong interest in growing a wide variety of sages, and one of the horticultural rules that applies to these diverse plants is that after a few years, they appreciate being dug up, divided at the crown, and replanted. I had grown *Salvia przewalskii* on a recommendation from another gardener, and the plants were truly worth it, making dense mounds topped by oversized flowers of bright blue. After a few years I dug one up to divide and transplant, and was immediately struck by the bright red color of the roots. After replanting, I got out my references to Chinese medicine, and found *S. przewalskii* listed as dan-shen gansu, one of the main alternative species for the production of medicinal danshen. Sometimes it's the books that lead you to the plants, but other times, it's the plants that lead you to the books!

Dang-gui (Dong-quai, Tang-kuei) (*Angelica sinensis*) Family: Carrot (*Apiaceae*)

Part used: Root dug during the fall of the second or third year of growth, dried and cured. Due to the tendency to rot, the roots are harvested during dry weather and shaken free of dirt (not washed). The roots may then be dried in the sun or dried slowly in the smoke of a wood fire to cure them. The roots are turned repeatedly or strung on a string, to afford even dehydration.

Tincture of dry root: 1:5 (50A:50W)
Dang-gui contains both alcohol-soluble volatile oils and water-soluble constituents that have opposite physiological effects on both blood pressure and uterine contractility. Therefore, equal quantities of water and alcohol are called for in this formula in order to help harmonize the action of the extract.

Water extracts: Basic tea or decoction. The tea of the ground root is generally preferred, as it captures some volatile constituents that are lost during the extended simmering called for in making a decoction.

Practical uses: Dang-gui tonifies, detoxifies, and nourishes the blood, while it improves peripheral circulation. The herb regulates the menstrual period and relaxes menstrual cramps, protects and nourishes the liver, helps arrest uterine bleeding, and is a gentle laxative best used to treat chronic constipation.

Dosage: According to basic recommendations found under "Dosage of tinctures," pages 49–52 and "Dosage of teas and decoctions," pages 70–71.

Contraindications: Not to be used during pregnancy. Not appropriate for patients with diarrhea.

Dang-shen (Codonopsis) (*Codonopsis pilosula*)
Family: Bellflower (*Campanulaceae*)

Part used: Root of 2-year or older plants dug during dormancy and used fresh or dried.

Tincture of fresh root: 1:2 (50A:50W)

Tincture of dried root: 1:5 (25A:75W)

Water extract: Decoction of fresh or dried root.

Practical uses: Dang-shen is used in much the same way as ginseng—to revitalize energy reserves, strengthen the immune system, and tonify the blood. Some of the many specific conditions assisted by daily use of this herb are asthma, anemia, exhaustion, gastroenteritis, indigestion, and diabetes.

Dosage: According to basic recommendations found under "Dosage of tinctures," pages 49–52 and "Dosage of teas and decoctions," pages 70–71.

Poultice: The fresh, pounded root and the soft, smooth, leaves of dang-shen are used in traditional Chinese medicine for poulticing, to speed healing and reduce inflammation of wounds and ulcerations.

Food use: The dried roots are powdered and added to cooked food. A large, fresh root can be split and added to soup, lending a celery-like flavor, often used in combination with astragalus and shiitake mushrooms. Fresh dang-shen root would make a sensible addition to the produce section of food stores worldwide.

Contraindications: None known. Safe for general use.

Other species: Sichuan dang-shen (*Codonopsis tangshen*) is similar in appearance to *C. pilosula* and is medicinally interchangeable.

Dill (*Anethum graveolens*)
Family: Carrot (*Apiaceae*)

Parts used: Leaf harvested prior to flowering and used fresh or dried, without the stems. Seed harvested at maturity and dried.

Tincture of seed: 1:4 (75A:25W)
The seeds may be ground up or bruised, soaked overnight in the menstruum, then briefly blended the following day and macerated in the usual manner.

Water extracts: Basic tea of dried seeds or leaves.

Direct consumption: Chewing the seeds after a meal will assist in efficient digestion, reduces oral bacteria, fights gum disease, and freshens the breath.

Practical uses: Dill is a stimulating aromatic carminative that assists in digestion. Taken during meals or directly afterwards, the herb will have an antispasmodic and gas-relieving action. Safe for young ones, the tea or tincture will help relieve infant colic and childhood stomachache. In treating colic, the dill may be taken by the mother and will pass through the milk to the baby. Dill also helps stimulate production of breast milk. High in vitamins A, C, and calcium, dill will help prevent and treat osteoporosis. The herb is anti-inflammatory and may reduce pain of rheumatoid arthritis. Dill is a traditional treatment for menstrual irregularities, urinary tract infection, and hiccups.

Dosage: According to basic recommendations found under "Dosage of tinctures," pages 49–52 and "Dosage of teas and decoctions," pages 70–71.

Food use: The leaves and seeds make a spicy addition to salads, pickles, cheeses, and cream sauce.

Contraindications: None known. Safe for general use.

Echinacea (Purple Coneflower)
(*Echinacea* spp.)
Family: Aster (*Asteraceae*)

Parts used: Whole root dug during dormancy and used fresh or dried. Leaves and flowers (without the stems) harvested at peak flower and used fresh or dried. The flower heads must be split before drying. Use snips. Seed harvested at maturity and dried.

Tincture of fresh root or leaves and flowers: 1:2 (75A:25W) Given that the herb contains water- and alcohol-soluble constituents, the menstruum for the tinctures is designed to extract both fractions. The water-soluble polysaccharides lend a sweet initial taste to good quality root, aerial parts, or to the extract. The alcohol-soluble alkylamides are responsible for the oral "buzzing" sensation experienced when tasting freshly harvested root, aerial portions, or a good quality extract. Echinacea contains oxygen-labile constituents; therefore, the dried herb does not last long in storage, and fresh preparations are generally preferred (see page 43).

Tincture of dried root, leaves, and/or flowers: 1:5 (50A:50W)

Tincture of seed: 1:5 (75A:25W)
The seeds may be ground up or bruised prior to the addition of the menstruum. The seed is particularly high in the alkylamide constituents.

Glycerite of fresh root, leaves, and/or flowers: 1:2 (100Gly)

Water extracts: Tea of dried leaves and flowers. Decoction of dried root.

Direct consumption: A small piece (1 to 2 g) of the fresh or recently dried root may be held in the mouth and slowly chewed. This is as effective as any fancy preparation, a practice that comes to us from the original American herbalists, the Native Americans.

Practical uses: The herb is an immune-stimulant that increases overall resistance to disease. Useful in treating the early phases of bacterial or viral infection, echinacea speeds resolution of colds, flu, and all kinds of upper respiratory infection. The herb makes an anti-inflammatory treatment for infected wounds, or the bites of reptiles and insects. Echinacea is also a potent sialagogue (promotes salivation). One good test for the freshness of herb or extract is how much it stimulates your spit.

Dosage: According to basic recommendations found under "Dosage of tinctures," pages 49–52 and "Dosage of teas and decoctions," pages 70–71. Also see "Dosage of glycerites," page 63.

Oil, salve, or cream: Make an infused herbal oil of the dried leaves and flowers, then proceed to make salve or cream according to the procedure found in "Chapter 10, Basic Formulas for Herbal Oils, Salves, and Creams." This is useful as a cosmetic skin toner, for treating wounds, and as an anti-inflammatory against stings and venomous bites.

Contraindications: Safe for general consumption, although rare allergic reactions have been recorded. The advisability of using immune-enhancing herbs for treating autoimmune diseases has been challenged.

Other species: There are nine species of *Echinacea* native to North America. *E. angustifolia* and *E. purpurea* are of proven efficacy, although local herbalists use local species interchangeably and with good results. When the cross-section of the roots of *Echinacea* show black markations, this is a sign of strong medicinal activity. These markations are composed of melanin, a naturally dark pigment produced by the plant in response to the presence of diverse gram-negative, endophytic bacteria. Echinacea is particularly rich in these microbes, which, when taken internally, stimulate production of antibodies that fight colds and flu. Since *E. angustifolia* contains a higher concentration of melanin than the other species, this would support the common opinion among herbalists that *E. angustifolia* is the strongest medicine. The root of this plant is also very rich in alkylamides. Although the specific role of alkylamides in immunostimulation is yet unclear, their presence appears to be a keystone marker for an effective extract. *E. purpurea* shows high concentrations of water-soluble polysaccharides, alcohol-soluble alkylamides, and caffeic acid derivatives in both root and aerial parts. *E. pallida* is generally considered to be weaker than *E. angustifolia* and *E. purpurea*, although the plant boasts an expanded array of another class of constituents known as poly-acetylenes. The root of *E. paradoxa* is chemically similar to that of *E. pallida*, but contains higher concentrations of the alky-lamides and less concentration of the polyacetylene constituents. The several other indigenous American *Echinacea* species (*E. atrorubens, E. levigata, E. sanguinea,* and *E. simulata*) have not been adequately studied, but they are likely candidates for use as effective medicines. *E. tennesseensis* is demonstrably rich in the alkylamide fraction and therefore is of particular promise.

Elderberry, Black (*Sambucus nigra*)
Family: Honeysuckle (*Caprifoliaceae*)

Parts used: Leaf harvested at any time during the growth cycle and used fresh. Flowers and pollen harvested in early flowering stage and used fresh or dried. Dry on paper to capture the pollen. Berries harvested at peak ripeness and used fresh or dried.

Tincture of dried flowers: 1:5 (50A:50W)

Tincture of fresh flowers: 1:2 (75A:25W)

Glycerite of dried berries (excellent!): 1:5 (60 Gly:40W)

Acetum of fresh buds and flowers: Pack the flowers in a crock or jar and cover with simmering hot apple cider vinegar. Cover and set aside overnight, then pour off through cheesecloth. This is a specific remedy for sore throat.

Water extract: Basic tea of dried flowers, taken hot or cold.

Syrup: Smash the fresh berries, press out the juice, and reduce on the back of the stove to a thick consistency, then preserve with an equal volume of honey or glycerine. The syrup can also be made by reconstituting dried berries. Follow the procedure found on pages 78–79, "Syrup made from reduced berries."

Practical uses: Elderberry flowers and berries are antiviral and immune-stimulating. When taken hot, the tea of elderberry flowers or elderberry tincture in hot water will help sweat out a cold or a fever. When taken cold, the tea is diuretic. Elderberry is commonly used for treating upper respiratory infection, including the common cold and flu. The berries are quite high in health-promoting procyanidins. The purple, blue, and black berries are best for direct consumption and for making syrup. The red berries are considered less choice. Don't eat the raw seed (see "Contraindications").

Dosage: According to recommendations found under "Dosage of tinctures," pages 49–52, "Dosage of glycerites," page 63, and "Dosage of teas and decoctions," pages 70–71. Dosage of elderberry fresh buds and flowers acetum is 1 tablespoonful (5 ml) taken up to 5 times per day.

External: The cooled tea of dried elderberry flowers is used as a wash or compress for improving oily skin or acne or for treating injured tissues. Similarly, you can dilute 2 droppersful of the tincture (60 drops) in 1 cup (240 ml) of cold water and use as a compress.

Bath or soak: The dried elderberry flowers are placed in a muslin bag, tied shut with string, and introduced into the hot bath or face wash. This is good for improving the tone of the skin. To sweat out a fever, the hot tea or the tincture in hot water is sipped, while one sits in the hot elder bath. Soak for 20 minutes, then wrap in a sheet and a blanket and go to bed. You will sweat.

Oil, salve, or cream: Make infused herbal oil of the fresh, green elderberry leaves. This can be used as-is or may be further processed into a delightfully cooling, green salve or cream. Follow the procedure described in "Chapter 10, Basic Formulas for Herbal Oils, Salves, and Creams" (see page 83). Oily preparations of fresh elder leaves make a useful treatment for traumatic injuries, old burns, ulcerations, or hemorrhoids.

Contraindications: The flowers of all the true elderberries are safe for general consumption, and the leaves are quite harmless for external use. The seeds in the berries can be toxic if taken raw, causing nausea and sometimes vomiting. The seeds of *Sambucus* species bearing red berries (e.g. *S. pubens, S. racemosa*) are most likely to prove toxic. The seeds of species bearing purple, blue, and black berries (e.g. *S. canadensis, S. caerulea and S. nigra*) are less likely to prove toxic. Cooking the berries reduces the toxicity of the seeds, but fresh berries need to be juiced and the seeds removed before consumption. Since the seeds provide no added medicinal advantage, it is recommended to exclude them from your finished product. The bark of root and stem are purgative and not recommended for internal use.

Other species: There are about 20 different species in the *Sambucus* genus found worldwide, all of which bear useful flowers and leaves. There are numerous cultivars of *S. canadensis,* mainly chosen for the production of large clusters of sweet berries. A few of the other significant species are Mexican elderberry (*S. mexicana*), blue elderberry (*S. caerulea*) of the western United States, Chinese elderberry (*S. javanica*), and the European dwarf elderberry (*S. ebulus*).

Elecampane (*Inula helenium*)
Family: Aster (*Asteraceae*)

Part used: Roots dug in the fall of the second or third year of growth. Allowed to grow older than this, the roots become woody and lose much of their medicinal potency. Roots may be used fresh, or sliced thinly and dried.

Tincture of fresh root: 1:2 (75A:25W)

Tincture of dried root: 1:5 (50A:50W)
The alcohol:water ratios for the tinctures of both fresh and dry roots are equilibrated in order to provide extraction of a balanced array of alcohol- and water-soluble constituents. The alcohol-soluble fraction includes antimicrobial essential oils, resins, and the antiparasitic molecule alantolactone, which is named "elecampane camphor" in the older texts. The water-soluble fraction is made up mainly of inulin, a mucilaginous polysaccharide molecule that can also be found in the roots of other members of the *Asteraceae,* including burdock and Jerusalem artichokes.

Water extract: Basic tea of dried roots. Decoction of dried roots. The water extracts are serviceable antitussives, actively representing the demulcent and nutritive aspects of the herb.

Syrup: Combine 1 part of the strong decoction with 2 parts of honey. Follow procedure found in "Chapter 9, Herbal Succi and Syrups," pages 77–78.

Honeyed roots: Wash, peel, and slice roots of elecampane, then simmer in honey according to the directions on page 80. The honeyed roots may be eaten as a lung or digestive tonic, or to allay coughing. They impart a glowing warmth to the chest. Eat the honey, too.

Practical uses: Elecampane is the premier treatment for acute or chronic disorders of the upper respiratory tract. It is gentle enough even for children. As a cough medicine, the herb is demulcent, antitussive, and expectorant—a specific for arresting irritable coughing when there is abundant expectoration. The herb also imparts a localized anesthetic influence to the tissues of the throat. As a treatment for upper respiratory tract infection, elecampane exerts a deep-seated antimicrobial influence—an excellent choice for treating viral, fungal, or bacterial infections, including staph. Elecampane has even been successful in treating tuberculosis. This is also one of the better herbs to use in treatment of humid bronchial asthma and associated shortness of breath. Elecampane is mildly bitter and highly nutritive, helping tonify the respiratory, digestive, and urinary organs, assisting in restoration of appetite and affording a rapid and complete recovery from illness. It is also a vermifuge, usually combined with other antiparasitic herbs, such as aloe, andrographis, black seed, and/or wormwood, in treatment of amoebic infestations, such as giardia (*Giardia lamblia*) and intestinal worms, such as roundworm (*Ascaris lumbricoides*).

Contraindications: Do not use if pregnant or nursing. Also, the pure essential oil of elecampane is best avoided, as it is likely to cause contact dermatitis due to the unmitigated concentration of irritating sesquiterpene lactones.

Other species: Inula is a genus of over 100 species of perennial plants belonging to the largest of all plant families, the *Asteraceae.* Some are impressive, such as magnificent elecampane *(Inula magnifica),* with its perfumed leaves and purple-black stems bearing clusters of radiant yellow flowers; others are weedy, growing in rocky, marginal areas or in saline soils at the seaside (e.g. the barely edible herb known as *I. crithmoides,* the golden samphire). *Inula britannica,* known commonly as British yellowhead, English elecampane, or meadow fleabane, is native to Asia and has been naturalized in Britain. The plant is used medicinally in much the same way as elecampane. The dried flowers of *Inula britannica* var. *chinensis* compose the Chinese herb xuan-fu-hua, which is classified as a warm herb that transfers phlegm/cold. *Inula conyza,* otherwise known as ploughman's spikenard or great fleabane, is native to Britain. There are marked similarities between this plant and *Inula viscosa,* the sticky fleabane. The highly aromatic aerial parts of both of these plants are used. The herb is burned and the ashes used as an insecticide. In antiquity, ploughman's spikenard was considered to be a good astringent for treating external wounds, bruising, and traumatic internal rupturing. *Inula graveolens* (syn. *Dittrichia graveolens, I. odorata),* known commonly as fragrant aster or sweet inula, is native to France and Corsica. Properly diluted, the volatile oil of this plant is used extensively in aromatherapy and is safe for external use, stimulating lymphatic drainage and circulation—an effective treatment for chronic lung problems and sinus congestion. *Inula royleana,* known commonly as Himalayan elecampane, is native to the western Himalayan mountains and Kashmir. The plant is antiparasitic and disinfectant, but is also potentially poisonous.

Eleuthero (Ci-wu-jia, "Siberian Ginseng") (*Eleutherococcus senticosus*) Family: Ginseng (*Araliaceae*)

Part used: The medicine consists of the rhizome (the root) dug in dormancy and used fresh or dried. The highest grade extracts employ the root bark only, whittled from the rhizome. Although the plant is common in its moist, cold, northern habititat, it is rare in cultivation. Therefore, it makes sense to harvest the roots without killing the plant. This may be accomplished by digging the running rhizome, which connects the parent plant from its ramet (offspring that occurs at a distance). The running rhizome is pencil thin, easy to dig, wash, and cut up, and makes excellent medicine. If the ramet becomes dislodged during this process, it may be gainfully re-planted.

Tincture of fresh root: 1:2 (75A:25W)

Tincture of dried root: 1:5 (50A:50W)

Water extracts: Basic decoction of the dried root.

Practical uses: Eleuthero helps one adapt to stress, whether it be emotional, physical, or environmental in nature. The herb is immune-enhancing and improves energy levels. It is specifically used by athletes to improve strength, stamina, and performance and is not classified as a stimulant or steroid. The herb also has a profound normalizing and balancing effect on blood pressure and blood sugar levels. A very important effect, shared also by astragalus, holy basil, and schisandra, is in protecting the body during radiation and chemotherapy, lessening side effects and improving overall energy and comfort.

Dosage: According to basic recommendations found under "Dosage of tinctures," pages 49–52 and "Dosage of teas and decoctions," pages 70–71. Best taken in the morning only.

Contraindications: Use of eleuthero is usually reserved for teenagers and adults. Overdose can cause sleeplessness, elevated blood pressure, and/or temporary flush or rash of the skin, usually occurring on the chest and neck. If these symptoms appear, reduce dosage, increase exercise, or discontinue use.

Eucalyptus
(*Eucalyptus* spp.)
Family: Myrtle (*Myrtaceae*)

Parts used: Fresh or dried leaves.

Tincture of dried leaves: 1:5 (100A)

Water extract: Basic tea of fresh or dried leaves, kept tightly covered during steeping to capture the volatile essential oils.

Practical uses: Eucalyptus is antiseptic to the upper respiratory tract and helps clear the sinuses. The steam arising from hot eucalyptus tea will also quickly clear clogged sinus passages.

Dosage: According to basic recommendations found under "Dosage of tinctures," pages 49–52 and "Dosage of teas and decoctions," pages 70–71. Always dilute the tincture in at least 1 cup (240 ml) of cold water before taking. See "Contraindications."

External: The tea or dilute tincture may be used as a gargle against sore throat or as a wash or compress for treating wounds and abrasions. Eucalyptus also make a credible insect repellent. Rub the fresh leaves on your body or dilute the essential oil in a neutral base (e.g. olive oil or jojoba oil) and apply to the skin. Here on the West Coast, when camping or hiking in the forest, if body lice, mosquitoes, or other insects disrupt the fun, then coming upon a grove of eucalyptus trees is considered to be a stroke of luck. After rubbing the leaves on one's body, a sort of nest may be made of the fallen leaves, and sleeping therein, one is protected from predation by small insects.

Contraindications: Not for use during pregnancy. Essential oil of eucalyptus contains large quantities of a molecule known as cineole, which is a recognized skin irritant. The pure essential oil should be used externally only, well-diluted before use by mixing in a neutral base, such as olive, apricot, or jojoba oil.

Other species: *Eucalyptus dives, E. globulus, E. nitens, E. oleosa, E. polybractea, E. radiata* and *E. smithii* are all particularly rich in essential oils and have been used in the herb industry for distilling the pure essential oil. The other 515 known species of the *Eucalyptus* genus are also medicinally active.

Evening Primrose (*Oenothera biennis*)
Family: Willowherb (*Onagraceae*)

Parts used: The entire fresh plant, including root and leaves, harvested in the first year and used fresh or dried. Flowers, seed pods and seeds harvested in the second year and used fresh or dried.

Tincture of entire fresh plant: 1:2 (50A:50W)

Tincture of dried plant: 1:5 (25A:75W)

Direct consumption: Evening primrose is an anti-inflammatory and nutritious herb that is at its best when employed as a food. The fresh root of young plants is delicious—sweet and spicy, and may be eaten fresh or used in stir-fry or soup. The leaves may be added to salads. They are agreeably mucilaginous and neutral in taste. The flowers are tasty and also rich in mucilage, making an excellent garnish for salads. The seeds may be sprinkled on food or used in salad dressings. They are about the size and texture of poppy seeds and are richly endowed with essential fatty acids.

Practical uses: Made into a tincture, the plant serves as a medicine for treating migraine, pelvic fullness, and other uncomfortable symptoms of PMS and menopause. Over time, use of evening primrose will impart lasting tone to the female reproductive organs. The herb is a gentle liver stimulant and slightly laxative, also containing a large amount of soothing mucilage. Evening primrose is therefore of use in treating indigestion—even when accompanied by diarrhea or vomiting.

Dosage: According to basic recommendations found under "Dosage of tinctures," pages 49–52.

Contraindications: The entire plant is safe to eat, but as with all wild foods, should not be consumed in excess and is best combined with other fare. Taking the plant alone and in excessive quantities is likely to *cause* gastric distress instead of *alleviating* it.

Other species: *Oenothera* is a genus represented by 80 species, many of them native to North America. Most of these are annuals, perennials, or recumbent plants. The best medicine comes from biennial, upright species such as *O. agrillucola, O. biennis, O. hookeri, O. longissima,* and *O. pilosella.*

𝓕

Fennel (*Foeniculum vulgare*)
Family: Carrot (*Apiaceae*)

Part used: Fresh, immature green seed or mature, dried seed.

Tincture of green or dried seed: 1:4 (75A:25W)
Bruise the seeds by grinding briefly in a blender, soak overnight in the menstruum, then blend the following morning and macerate in the usual manner.

Glycerite of fresh green seed: 1:3 (100Gly)
The seeds can be soaked overnight in the glycerin, then briefly blended the following day and macerated in the usual manner.

Water extracts: Tea of seed (or tea of bruised seed—stronger).

Direct consumption: Chew the seed.

Practical uses: Fennel is a good digestive herb, generally added to dishes containing meat or cheese or taken after the meal to freshen the breath, improve assimilation of food, and decrease gas. The tincture or tea synergizes well with laxatives, acting as an antispasmodic. Fennel is also an acceptable flavoring agent for bitter medicines. The herb is completely safe for infants and will almost always relieve colic when administered as a weak tea by the teaspoonful (5 ml). Alternately, the mother can take the extract or drink the tea. Not only does this improve digestibility of the mother's milk, but it also stimulates letdown reflex and improves milk production. Infant colic is usually a reaction to an allergen in the mother's diet (such as wheat gluten or dairy products), so it makes sense to observe what foods might be causing the problem, in order to nip it, so to speak, in the bud.

Dosage: According to basic recommendations found under "Dosage of tinctures," pages 49–52 and "Dosage of teas and decoctions," pages 70–71. Also see "Dosage of glycerites," page 63.

Contraindications: Large amounts not to be taken during pregnancy.

Feverfew (*Tanacetum parthenium*)
Family: Aster (*Asteraceae*)

Parts used: Leaf and flower harvested at peak flower, removed from the stem, and used fresh or dried.

Tincture of fresh herb: 1:2 (75A:25W)

Tincture of recently dried herb: 1:5 (50A:50W)

Water extract: Basic tea.

Direct consumption: The leaves may be taken sparingly in salads or on a bread-and-butter sandwich. This is for the medicinal (not culinary) effect.

Practical uses: Feverfew is a good nervine tonic with specific application against migraine and low spirits. Part of its anti-migraine effect is due to anti-inflammatory activity and part due to the positive bitter digestive effects.

Dosage: According to basic recommendations found under "Dosage of tinctures," pages 49–52 and "Dosage of teas and decoctions," pages 70–71. The antimigraine effect is best accomplished by taking a small amount of the herb on a daily basis, not by taking large amounts of the herb during the actual episode, although this does work for some people.

Contraindications: Not to be used during pregnancy. Rare adverse reactions have been recorded.

Figwort (*Scrophularia nodosa*)
Family: Figwort (*Scrophulariaceae*)

Parts used: Leaves and/or root harvested prior to seeding stage and used fresh or dried.

Tincture of fresh herb or root: 1:2 (75A:25W)

Water extract: Basic tea or decoction of the dried leaves or root.

Practical uses: Figwort is a lymphatic stimulant, and has been used for treating congestion in the lymph nodes and lymphatic cancer. The herb is also a general anti-inflammatory, having shown some promise in treating arthritis and eczema.

Dosage: Internally, figwort is best taken in combination with other alterative and cleansing herbs such as burdock, yellow dock, red clover, and/or dandelion. The dosage of figwort tincture is 5 to 15 drops in 1 cup of water, 3 to 5 times daily.

External: The full-strength decoction or 1 dropperful of the tincture diluted in 1 cup of hot water make an external application for treating wounds, ulcerations, swellings, abrasions, and contusions. This is best applied as a hot compress, allowing the injured area to air dry between treatments.

Poultice: The fresh leaves are bruised or mashed and laid directly on the skin. This is a good treatment for wounds, tenacious sores, burns, infections, or blood poisoning. Given the widespread distribution of the easily-identified figworts, hikers of the wild country would be well-advised to understand the first aid potential of the poultice of this plant.

Oil, salve, or cream: Make infused herbal oil of the fresh leaves. This can be used as-is or as an ingredient for making salve or cream according to the procedure found in "Chapter 10, Basic Formulas for Herbal Oils, Salves, and Creams," page 83, also pages 87–90. The oily preparations good for swollen lymph nodes, tumors, old burns, ulcerations, wounds, and abrasions.

Contraindications: Not to be used during pregnancy. The externally applied poultice and oily extracts are safe for general use. For internal use, seek the advice and care of a qualified health professional. Given the content of potentially cardioactive glycosides, figwort should not be taken in combination with heart medications or by those suffering from heart disease or cardiac irregularities.

Other species: There are about 200 species in the *Scrophularia* genus, many of which have been used by native peoples for poulticing and for the alterative effects. Common figwort (*S. nodosa*) from Europe is generally considered to be official, but indigenous American herbs are used interchangeably. These include carpenter's square (*S. marilandica*) of the east coast, California figwort (*S. californica)* of the western coastline, and lance-leaf figwort (*S. lanceolata*) which is widely distributed.

G

Garlic (*Allium sativum*)
Family: Lily (*Liliaceae*)

Part used: The cloves are fall-planted and the bulbs are harvested when mature, usually in midsummer or fall, when the ground is dry. The bulbs are broken apart to reveal the cloves, which are used fresh or cooked.

Tincture of fresh cloves: 1:2 (100A)
The cloves are crushed, then covered with grain alcohol. It is best not to blend into a mush or to remove the skins, because they provide a matrix for the menstruum to make its way around and through the sticky flesh of the garlic. Shake well to incorporate, then macerate, press, and filter in the usual manner.

Direct consumption: Raw versus cooked garlic have different, but somewhat overlapping, effects. I generally recommend raw garlic for treating bacterial infections. Cooked garlic has a more deep-seated digestive and immune-enhancing effect. The cooked garlic is also preventative of arteriosclerosis (hardening of the arterial walls) and is used to help prevent and cure heart disease and many types of cancer.

Practical uses: Consuming garlic helps in the digestion of fats by increasing secretion of bile. The herb deeply affects the blood and the circulation, demonstrating fibrolinic (blood-thinning), antitumor, and anti-blood-cholesterol activity. The raw cloves, garlic oil, and tincture contain thiosulfinate compounds that exhibit marked antibacterial effect.

Dosage of tincture: According to basic recommendations found under "Dosage of tinctures," pages 49–52. See "Contraindications."

Cough formula: Crush 6 cloves of garlic, remove the skins, then put them into 1 cup (240 ml) of goat's milk in a saucepan and simmer until the garlic is tender. Add 1 tablespoon (15 ml) honey and take the thick liquid freely for the nutritive, immune-enhancing, antibiotic, expectorant, and cough-suppressing effects. The stout of heart may also wish to eat the barely cooked garlic.

Garlic ear oil: Combine 1 part by weight of the fresh, crushed cloves of garlic with 1 part by weight of fresh mullein flowers. Do not remove the skins from the garlic, as they prevent the mass from balling up, which keeps it from rotting during the extraction. Immediately combine this herbal mixture (garlic and mullein flowers) with olive oil in a gallon jar at the concentration of 1 part weight of fresh herbal mixture in g:1 part volume of olive oil in ml. Stir the herb and oil mixture thoroughly, cover the mouth of the jar with cheesecloth, and set it in the sunshine to macerate for 3 or more days. The oil needs to completely cover the infusing herbs. It is important not to cook the oil with artificial heat, instead allowing the sunlight to slowly fuel the process of extraction. High temperatures degrade the antibiotic compounds that are so effective in treating inner ear infection. At the end of 3 days, gently express the macerating extract through multiple layers of cheesecloth. This is done by hand or if using an herb press, by exerting only minimal pressure. Collect the resultant herb-infused oil in a jar and set aside to settle overnight. Water and garlic juice will sink to the bottom of the jar. In the morning, decant the pure oil through several layers of clean, dry cheesecloth, leaving the watery sludge behind. The finished oil must not contain water droplets. Properly label and store the oil in amber bottles, tightly stoppered, in a cool, dark place. Oil made in this manner will retain its goodness for at least a year. The dosage of ear oil is 1 drop per ear, 1 to 3 times daily. Warm the oil to body temperature before application. Flooding the ear with oil does not improve the effect and is not recommended. Massaging the soft tissues behind the ear lobe with the warmed ear oil, however, is absolutely recommended.

Contraindications: Nursing mothers should know that the garlic goes through the milk and is sometimes responsible for causing gastric upset in nursing babies. The odor of garlic will pervade the breath and the skin. High dosage of raw garlic or garlic tincture may cause gastrointestinal disturbance, nausea, and sometimes vomiting in predisposed individuals. Administering garlic tincture in milk, as opposed to water, will provide an emollient effect that subdues side effects.

Gentian, Yellow (*Gentiana lutea*)
Family: Gentian (*Gentianaceae*)

Parts used: Root and rhizome (the root) dug during dormancy and used fresh or dried. Although the aerial parts (leaves and stems) of the plant are not traditionally used, they are intensely bitter and may be substituted for the root. It is nice to make the medicine without sacrificing the life of the plant!

Tincture of fresh root or aerial parts: 1:2 (75A:25W)

Tincture of dried root or aerial parts: 1:5 (50A:50W)

Water extracts: Cold infusion. Basic tea or decoction of fresh or dried root or aerial parts.

Direct consumption: Chew a small piece of the fresh leaf or root.

Practical uses: Gentian is the purest of bitter tonics, directly stimulating the salivary and gastric secretions. The herb acts to improve appetite, reduce acid indigestion, and tonify the digestive tract.

Dosage: According to basic recommendations found under "Dosage of tinctures," pages 49–52 and "Dosage of teas and decoctions," pages 70–71. Best taken just prior to meals.

Contraindications: Do not take if suffering from gastric or duodenal ulcer or inflammation of the gastrointestinal tract. Predisposed individuals may experience headache when taking gentian, especially on an empty stomach. If this occurs, take during meals, not prior to meals.

Other species: Several other herbs in the gentian family are nontoxic and medicinally interchangeable with yellow gentian. These include Tibetan gentian (*G. tibetica*), and the various indigenous American *Gentiana* species (e.g. *G. affinis*, *G. alba*, *G. andrewsii*, *G. austromontana*, *G. bisetaea*, *G. calycosa*, *G. clausa*, *G. decora*, *G. newberryi*, *G. saponaria*, and *G. villosa*). Gentian species are protected throughout most of their native range. These plants are sensitive, rare, and must never be taken from the wild. They can be very successfully cultivated from seed.

179

Ginseng, American (*Panax quinquefolius*)
Family: Ginseng (*Araliaceae*)

Part used: Root harvested in the fall after maturation of the fruit and seed, used fresh or dried. Ginseng is not imbued with its full medicinal potential until the roots reach 7 years of age. However, the roots are often dug and utilized after the third year of growth and exhibit some activity even at this immature stage. Roots cultivated in a hardwood forest are preferred over those grown under shade cloth.

Tincture of fresh root: 1:2 (75A:25W)

Tincture of dried root: 1:5 (50A:50W)

Glycerite of fresh root: 1:2 (100Gly)

Direct consumption: Chew the fresh or dried root. The dosage is about 1 g of the dry or 3 g of the fresh root per day for the adaptogenic effects. Greater quantities will stimulate the central nervous system and often prove markedly aphrodisiacal.

Practical uses: Ginseng is adaptogenic, helping one cope with stress, whether caused by emotional, physical, or environmental factors. The herb boosts energy, improves work performance, increases resistance to disease, tonifies nerves, improves sexual stamina and potency, has a normalizing effect (reduces high blood sugar and cholesterol, increases low red blood cell count, raises low blood pressure, lowers high blood pressure), is a digestive tonic, protects from the deleterious effects of radiation and chemotherapy, and promotes longevity.

Dosage: According to basic recommendations found under "Dosage of tinctures," pages 49–52 and "Dosage of teas and decoctions," pages 70–71. Also see "Dosage of glycerites", page 63.

Contraindications: Use of ginseng is usually reserved for teen-agers and adults. May cause sleeplessness if taken in the evening. Not to be taken by those suffering from acute-phase inflammatory conditions, such as colds, flu, and fevers. Popular opinion that ginseng is exclusively for men is a myth.

Other species: Chinese or Asian ginseng (*Panax ginseng*) is for all practical purposes medicinally interchangeable with American ginseng (*P. quinquefolius*). Eleuthero (*Eleutherococcus senticosus*) and Rhodiola (*Rhodiola rosea*) are also employed as adaptogens and ginseng substitutes. American dwarf ginseng (*Panax trifolius*) is too small to be practical. See "Eleuthero," "Rhodiola," and "Spikenard."

Goldenrod (*Solidago canadensis*)
Family: Aster (*Asteraceae*)

Parts used: Leaves and flowers harvested in the early flowering stage, without the stem.

Tincture of fresh herb: 1:2 (75A:25W)

Tincture of dried herb: 1:5 (50A:50W)

Water extracts: Cold infusion. Basic tea of dried herb. Hot tea will cause sweating. Warm or cold tea will act as a diuretic, for treatment of urinary infection.

Practical uses: Goldenrod is a soothing tonic for the entire genito-urinary tract. The herb is useful as a diuretic and antiseptic for treating kidney or bladder infection.

Dosage: According to basic recommendations found under "Dosage of tinctures," pages 49–52 and "Dosage of teas and decoctions," pages 70–71.

Contraindications: None known. Safe for general use. Purported allergies to goldenrod are usually attributable to ragweeds (*Ambrosia spp.*), which bloom simultaneously. When processing dried goldenrod flowers, the use of a filter mask is recommended due to the presence of tiny, airborne particles.

Other species: The *Solidago* genus consists of about 130 species, many of which are useful medicinals. Early goldenrod (*S. gigantea*), Canada goldenrod (*S. canadensis*), sweet goldenrod (*S. odora*), and European goldenrod (*S. virgaurea*) are used interchangeably and are all characterized by the bright yellow, flowering plume and delightfully delicate fragrance.

181

Goldenseal (*Hydrastis canadensis*)
Family: Crowfoot (*Ranunculaceae*)

Parts used: Root and rhizome (the root) dug from autumn to spring, used fresh or dried. Leaf and stem harvested after the plant has gone to seed, used fresh or dried. Combining the roots and aerial parts (leaves and stems) prior to extraction will produce a more effective tincture. This includes the efflux pump inhibitors that reside in the aerial parts of the plant, which synergize with the root alkaloids to disarm gram-positive bacteria. Use 4 parts by weight root to 1 part by weight aerial parts.

Tincture of fresh root (with leaf if possible): 1:2 (75A:25W)

Tincture of dried root (with leaf if possible): 1:5 (50A:50W) Equal parts of water and alcohol are used because isoquinoline alkaloids are both water- and alcohol-soluble.

Water extract: Basic tea or cold infusion of dried leaf and stem or a cold infusion made by mixing ½ teaspoon of dried, powdered root in 1 cup of cold, distilled water (equivalent to 1 g of powder in 240 ml of cold, distilled water). Used externally, this becomes an astringent and antibacterial wash.

Practical uses: Goldenseal is antimicrobial and tonifies the mucous membranes. The herb is often inappropriately used at the first signs of upper respiratory infection and is best employed during second-phase upper-respiratory infections where there is redness and swelling of the membranes and/or copious discharge of thick yellow or green mucous. Naturopaths commonly use goldenseal in combination with Echinacea, myrrh, and minute doses of poke for treating streptococcal infections of the tonsils. In small doses, Goldenseal acts as a bitter stimulant to the digestion and tonifies the entire digestive tract. The value of using goldenseal as an antiparasitic and as an alterative for treating cancer should not be overlooked. The herb is a gynecological remedy for controlling uterine bleeding.

Dosage: According to basic recommendations found under "Dosage of tinctures," pages 49–52 and "Dosage of teas and decoctions," pages 70–71. The tincture of leaf and stem contains the same constituents (the alkaloids berberine and hydrastine) as the root, but in lesser concentration. Therefore, the dosage of products made with leaf and stem may have to be doubled or tripled to achieve the same effect. As previously mentioned, combining both the root and the leaves produces a more reliable antibacterial medicine. As a digestive bitter, the tea of aerial parts is recommended to be sipped just before eating.

Oil, salve, or cream: Make infused herbal oil of the fresh or dried leaves and stems of goldenseal along with other ingredients such as calendula flowers, chickweed, and comfrey. This oil may be further processed into salve or cream (see "Chapter 10, Basic Formulas for Herbal Oils, Salves, and Creams," pages 81–90). These products have an antibacterial effect, and are especially healing to mucous membranes. Another method of making goldenseal salve is to stir the dried, finely powdered root into a sticky base, such as lanolin, or into finished herbal salve.

External: The powder of root and rhizome may be dusted directly on wounds as an antibacterial dressing. The tincture may be applied full-strength or diluted at the rate of 1 dropperful (30 drops) per cup (240 ml) of cold water for treating infected wounds, eczema, hemorrhoids, and skin ulcerations. The salve made from the infused herbal oil may be similarly employed.

Eye wash for treating conjunctivitis (pinkeye): Combine in a clean glass 1 cup (240 ml) of distilled water and ¼ teaspoon of table salt, swirling well to dissolve. This isotonic solution balances the salinity with that of the human body, which makes the wash more soothing to the eyes. Add 10 drops of goldenseal tincture to this isotonic solution and bathe the eyes, either by using a clean dropper, a sterile eyecup, or a compress. Treat the eyes several times daily until symptoms disappear. Make the eye wash fresh daily.

Nasal douche for treating sinusitis: 30 drops of the root tincture diluted in ½ cup of isotonic water, twice daily. Cold infusion of dried root used full strength, twice daily. Put the solution in your cupped hand and snort it up your nose. A less heroic method, is to gargle, tilting the head back and working the jaw to introduce the solution into the sinuses. Taking the tincture internally at prescribed dosage is a helpful adjunct therapy.

Douche for treating leukorrhea (white vaginal discharge): 30 drops of the root tincture in 2 cups of warm water, twice daily. Cold infusion of dried root used full strength, twice daily.

Contraindications: Internal use is not recommended during pregnancy or for those suffering from elevated blood pressure. Extended use on mucous membranes may cause excessive dryness.

Other species: Potential substitutes for goldenseal are other berberine-rich medicinals, such as goldthread (*Coptis* spp.) and Oregon grape (*Mahonia* spp.). Even yerba mansa (*Anemopsis californica*), twinleaf (*Jeffersonia diphylla*), and Baical skullcap (*Scutellaria baicalensis*), which contain little or no berberine, have been proposed as substitutes, due to their anti-bacterial effects. Although all of these plants can be used instead of goldenseal for some conditions, there is no direct substitute for true cultivated goldenseal, which contains a unique array of isoquinoline alkaloids, is respected worldwide, and occupies a special place in the hearts of American herbalists.

Goldthread (Huang-lian, Chinese Coptis)
(*Coptis chinensis*)
Family: Crowfoot (*Ranunculaceae*)

Parts used: The root and rhizome, dug from autumn to spring. Gently shake the roots to remove as much soil as possible, then briefly wash them in cold water. Lay the roots out to dry on screens in the shade and turn frequently. Once the tangled mass becomes fairly dry, transfer to a screen lined with paper, thereby saving any rootlets that might break off. Every little bit is good medicine! The root is best ground to a medium-fine powder prior to extraction.

Tincture of dry root: 1:5 (50A:50W) Because goldthread root is used at low dosage and is generally in short supply, tincturing (as opposed to decocting) is the most economical form of extraction. Equal parts of water and alcohol are used because isoquinoline alkaloids are both water- and alcohol-soluble.

Water extracts: The cold infusion is made by mixing ¼ teaspoon of dried, powdered root in 1 cup of cold, distilled water (equal to

0.5 g of powder in 240 ml of cold, distilled water). Alternatively, dispense 5 drops of goldthread tincture into 1 glass of water. Used externally, this becomes an astringent and antibacterial wash or compress for treating wounds and infections.

Practical uses (external): The water extract of goldthread may be used as an oral swish and gargle in treatment of inflamed mucous membranes of the mouth (stomatitis), including general redness and swelling, heavily coated tongue, periodontal disease, canker sores, other oral lesions, and sore throat. Goldthread may also be used in treating streptococcal infections of the tonsils, often in combination with Echinacea, myrrh, and poke.

Eye wash for treating conjunctivitis (pinkeye): Combine in a clean glass 1 cup (240 ml) of distilled water and ¼ teaspoon of table salt, swirling well to dissolve. This isotonic solution balances the salinity with that of the human body, which makes the wash more soothing to the eyes. Add 5 drops of goldthread tincture to this isotonic solution and bathe the eyes, either by using a clean dropper, a sterile eyecup, or a compress. Treat the eyes several times daily until symptoms disappear. Make the eye wash fresh every day.

Practical uses (internal): In terms of traditional Chinese medicine, this is one of the herbs that clears heat, as it demonstrates bitter, cold, and drying properties. Goldthread is best combined with other herbs that help balance its powerful influence and direct its activity toward the relevant body organs. Probably the most important action of this herb is its ability to combat diarrhea, dysentery, high fever, and other symptoms of contagion caused by harmful bacteria. Used in this way, often in combination with Baical skullcap (*Scutellaria baicalensis*), goldthread is really an unparalleled treatment—diarrhea abates, stomach pain diminishes, and digestion is normalized.

Dosage (internal): For moderate symptoms of stomach upset or indigestion, take 1 to 5 drops of the tincture, 3 times daily, just prior to meals, diluted in at least ½ glass of water. For acute bacterial dysentery, increase dosage to 10 drops up to 5 times daily, diluted in at least ½ glass of water.

Contraindications: Not to be taken by pregnant or nursing women. Not to be used by infants or small children. Not to be taken by those suffering from problems with the gall bladder. Generally well-suited to teenagers and adults. The herb is intensely bitter, and if taking it causes nausea, then follow it up with a food that is high in soluble fiber. Fresh blueberries or bilberries will prove antinauseant, as will oatmeal water. To make oatmeal water, stir 1 heaping tablespoon of fine oatmeal (*Avena sativa*) into a glass of water. The high soluble fiber nourishes the intestinal membranes and ameliorates nausea.

Other species: Coptis is a genus of at least 10 species, which include representatives native to both Asia and America. Huang-lian (*C. chinensis*) is the most root-productive of all, and therefore supplies much of the world demand. The American species are *C. groenlandica* in the east, and *C. occidentalis* in the west. They produce rootlets that are truly threadlike and are low yielding, but they are medicinally just as strong as the medicines from Asia, and may be used interchangeably.

Gotu Kola (*Centella asiatica* syn. *Hydrocotyl asiatica*)
Family: Carrot (*Apiaceae*)

Parts used: Whole herb, with or without the root, used fresh or dried.

Tincture of fresh herb: 1:2 (75A:25W)

Tincture of dried herb: 1:5 (50A:50W)

Water extract: Tea of fresh or dried herb.

Succus of fresh herb: 1 part alcohol by volume: 3 parts gotu kola juice by volume (see "Chapter 9, Herbal Succi and Syrups").

Direct consumption: Chew and eat the young, fresh leaves.

Practical uses: In Ayurvedic medicine, gotu kola is considered to be a rejuvenating tonic to the life force and to the memory. The herb stimulates rapid and healthy growth of hair, skin, and nails. Gotu kola speeds healing of wounds, hyperextended joints and stretched or injured ligaments, and improves vascular health.

Dosage: According to basic recommendations found under "Dosage of tinctures," pages 49–52 and "Dosage of teas and decoctions," pages 70–71.

Poultice: The fresh leaves are bruised or mashed and applied to wounds, contusions, swellings, or oily skin. This speeds healing, reduces formation of scar tissue, and rejuvenates the tissues.

Oil, salve, or cream: Make infused herbal oil of the fresh or dried leaf and stem of gotu kola. This can be used as-is or can be further processed into salve or cream according to the procedure found in "Chapter 10, Basic Formulas for Herbal Oils, Salves, and Creams." The oily preparations of gotu kola are used for healing and rejuvenating the skin and hair.

Food use: Fresh young gotu kola leaves are excellent in salads, but the older leaves can be quite bitter. The fresh leaves are juiced, diluted with 2 parts of water, and sweetened to make a healthy, green drink. The leaves can also be added to stir-fry and soup.

Contraindications: None known. Safe for general use.

Other species: Brahmi (*Bacopa monnieri*) has sometimes been confused with gotu kola, due to the similarity of their growth habit, the shared memory-enhancing activity, and because many Ayurvedic practitioners call gotu kola "brahmi." In this case, using the Latin names definitely dispels confusion. Gotu kola is a pantropical plant. Given this wide distribution, it is not surprising that several different strains with slightly different botanical characteristics have evolved in the tropics of the Old World, the New World, and on the various tropical islands. Practitioners may indicate a preference for one strain over another, but really, gotu kola is gotu kola is gotu kola.

Gravel Root (Joe Pye Weed, Queen-of-the-Meadow) (*Eupatorium purpureum*) Family: Aster (*Asteraceae*)

Part used: Root and rhizome (the root) harvested in dormancy, and used fresh or dried.

Tincture of the fresh root: 1:2 (75A:25W)

Tincture of the dried root: 1:5 (50A:50W)

Water extracts: Basic tea of ground, dried root. Basic decoction of the dried root.

Practical uses: Gravel root tonifies and cleanses the mucous membranes of the genito-urinary tract. The herb is helpful in treating cases of urinary stone and helps reverse prostatitis.

Dosage: According to basic recommendations found under "Dosage of tinctures," pages 49–52 and "Dosage of teas and decoctions," pages 70–71.

Contraindications: The aerial parts contain PAs, but the root contains little or none of these potentially liver-toxic substances. The root tends to move toxic substances *out* and not hold them. This time, I guess they got stuck in the leaves! On the basis of possible PA content, this plant should be avoided during pregnancy and should not be used by those suffering from liver disease.

Other species: The most direct substitute for gravel root is clearly the closely allied spotted Joe Pye weed (*Eupatorium maculatum*), which, for all practical purposes, may be used interchangeably. Gravel root, boneset (*E. perfoliatum*), hemp agrimony (*E. cannibinum*), and spotted Joe Pye weed all contain immune-stimulating polysaccharides. There are over 40 other species in the *Eupatorium* genus found worldwide and many of them are considered medicinal, including the indigenous American herb wild horehound (*E. aromaticum*), the Mexican-American herb mata (*E. herbacea*), and the Vietnamese herb man turoi (*E. staechadosmum*). See "Boneset."

188

Gumweed (Grindelia) (*Grindelia robusta*)
Family: Aster (*Asteraceae*)

Parts used: Leaves and flowers harvested in hot weather at the peak of flowering, without the stems. Grindelia flowers tend to stick together during processing, but nonetheless should be laid out thinly on the screens and turned frequently to dry.

Tincture of dried herb: 1:5 (100A) The high alcohol content helps dissolve the resins and makes a potent tincture. It is best to freeze the dried flowers overnight before grinding, to make them less likely to gum-up the grinder. Another option is to put the weighed flowers in a blender, cover with the alcohol, allow to sit overnight, then in the morning blend to completion, pour into a glass jar, macerate and press in the usual manner.

Practical uses: Gumweed relaxes and tonifies the mucous membranes of the upper respiratory tract. The herb is specifically indicated for treating chronic asthma and emphysema.

Dosage: According to basic recommendations found under "Dosage of tinctures," pages 49–52 and "Dosage of teas and decoctions," pages 70–71.

External: The tincture may be used full-strength as a topical dressing for insect bites, stings, and especially the rashes caused by poison ivy or poison oak. A good trailside remedy is to simply rub the flower on the affected area. Grindelia has a pain-relieving, drying, protective, and healing influence. The herb may be used as a medicinal ingredient in soap.

Contraindications: Large internal doses of gumweed can cause gastric or kidney irritation in predisposed individuals. If this occurs, reduce dosage or discontinue use.

Other species: The genus *Grindelia* is represented by over 50 different species, many of which have leaves that are glossy with resin and flower bracts full of white exudate. Besides *G. robusta,* a few of the medicinally useful species are *G. camporum, G. integrifolia, G. squarrosa and G. stricta.*

189

Hawthorn (*Crataegus monogyna, C. oxyacantha*)
Family: Rose (*Rosaceae*)

Parts used: Leaves and flowers harvested in the early flowering stage in the spring and used fresh or dried. Berries harvested when mature, after the first frost, used fresh or dried.

Tincture of fresh leaf and flower or fresh berries: 1:2 (75A:15W:10Gly)
The tincture of fresh hawthorn berries is problematical due to the high pectin content—the smashed berries clump together, and the finished tincture is very prone to precipitation.

Tincture of dried leaf and flower or dried berries: 1:5 (50A:40W:10Gly)
The dried berries are ground up, including the stone. Constituents in the stone are cardiotonic, and stone fragments break up the mash, improving maceration and yield.

Water extracts: Basic tea of dried leaf and flower or dried berries. Decoction of the dried berries.

Direct consumption: The fresh berries are delicious and may be used in season to fortify the heart—probably the mildest way to take the herb. Chew 6 or 7 berries a day and spit out the stones.

Syrup: Made by combining 1 part by volume of the strong decoction of the dried berries:2 parts by volume of honey (see "Chapter 9, Herbal Succi and Syrups," pages 76–9).

Practical uses: This is the premier herb for treating heart-related illness. Hawthorn is commonly and effectively used on an ongoing basis in recuperation from heart surgery or heart attack and for treating degenerative heart disease, arteriosclerosis, weakness of the heart muscle, and irregular heart beat. The herb regulates blood pressure and promotes a general sense of open-hearted well-being.

Dosage: According to basic recommendations found under "Dosage of tinctures," pages 49–52 and "Dosage of teas and decoctions," pages 70–71.

Food use: The dried berries can be made into an excellent jam that preserves the heart tonic properties of the herb.

Contraindications: Hawthorn may potentiate the effects of digitalis-based drugs, such as digoxin, and should not be taken concurrently with any pharmaceutical heart medicines.

Other species: Species in the *Crataegus* genus readily cross, so there is considerable variation of form. Wild hawthorns, including the American *C. monogyna* and the European *C. oxyacantha* (also known as *C. laevigata*) are considered official. Given the lack of comparative studies to demonstrate interchangeability of the leaves, flowers, and fruits of hybrid cultivars with the official species, I do not recommend using hybridized hawthorns (e.g. *C. monogyna* "autumn glory," *C. monogyna* "toba," and *C. lavellei*) for medicinal application. If the berry contains two or fewer seeds, it is probably a wild-form hawthorn. If it contains more than two seeds, it is probably a cultivated strain.

Helichrysum (*Helichrysum italicum*)
Family: Aster (*Asteraceae*)

Part used: Fresh or dried flowers, harvested in very early flowering stage and shade dried on screens. The flowers will tend to further mature and fluff during dehydration, and may need to be covered with a top screen to keep the fan or the wind from blowing them away. For tea use, whole, dried flowers are employed. For tincturing and infused oil, the dried flowers are first ground to a medium powder. For fresh tincture, the flowers are blended with the menstruum. For essential oil manufacture, the whole, fresh or dried flowers are packed in the still pot or alembic, and steam distilled.

Tincture of dried flowers: 1:5 (75A:25W)

Tincture of fresh flowers: 1:3 (100A)

Water extract: Basic tea of the dried flowers.

Oil, salve, or cream: Make infused herbal oil of the ground, dried flowers. This can be used as-is or may be further processed into salve or cream (see "Chapter 10, Basic Formulas for Herbal Oils, Salves, and Creams," pages 85–90).

Practical uses, external (essential oil or infused oil): Helichrysum essential oil is the most popular preparation. Although this is one of the safest essential oils to use directly on the skin, prudence calls for dilution, best achieved by mixing 2 to 5 drops of essential oil into 1 teaspoon of carrier oil (apricot kernel oil, rosehip seed oil, olive oil, jojoba oil, etc). The infused oil can easily be made at home, and may be used full-strength in therapy just as one would use the diluted essential oil. In either form, helichrysum may be used as a first aid treatment for resolving swelling, discoloration, and pain associated with bruises and sprains, as a massage oil to relieve muscle aches and pains or to appease arthritic joints, as a general circulatory stimulant for treating varicose veins and thrombosis, and as an application to the sensitive tissue behind the ears for treating hearing loss and tinnitus. The herb is a valuable astringent, anti-inflammatory, and cell proliferant—speeds healing of wounds and reduces formation of scar tissue; firms, strengthens and removes wrinkles in anti-aging therapy; helps erase stretch marks associated with pregnancy and lactation.

Practical uses, internal (tea or tincture): Helichrysum flowers are often used in tea mixtures where their bright color, lift, and aroma truly augment the blend. For instance, they are an ingredient in the *Unani* preparation known as *zahraa,* a formula that includes helichrysum, mallow, horsetail, mint, rose buds, sage, and dried black elderberries. Taken before meals, the tea or tincture of helichrysum alone will help improve appetite, reducing symptoms of poor digestion, nausea, and peptic ulcer. The herb stimulates the liver to increase output of bile, which helps in the assimilation of dietary fats (choleretic effect). Taken internally, helichrysum proves to be a good antibacterial and diuretic, for treating symptoms of urinary tract infection, swelling of extremities, and water retention.

Dosage: According to basic recommendations found under "Dosage of tinctures," pages 49–52 and "Dosage of teas and decoctions," pages 70–71.

Contraindications: Individuals with known allergies to plants in the *Aster* family should steer clear of this herb. For centuries Helichrysum has been used by countless cooks of Mediterranean cuisine, without incident, as a spice that mimics curry, which attests well to its overall safety and deliciousness. Furthermore, it is one of the few essential oils (along with essential oil of lavender) that is generally listed as safe for direct application to the skin.

Other species: There are over 500 closely allied species in the *Helichrysum* genus, many of them used locally in food and medicine. Of these, our *Helichrysum italicum* is the most famous, and manufacturers of essential oil seek this species in particular. The best plants will produce an oil that is high in azulene, a blue-colored sesquiterpene that lends a delightful aroma and a profound anti-inflammatory and antibacterial influence to the embrocation. Another species of note is immortelle (*H. arenarium*), which produces a medicinal tea for treatment of poor digestion and arthritis.

He-shou-wu (Ho-shou-wu, Fo-ti)
(*Polygonum multiflorum*)
Family: Knotweed (*Polygonaceae*)

Part used: Tuberous roots harvested in the fall of the third or fourth year of growth and used without further processing or processed in accordance with traditional Chinese methods.

Drying method: The tuberous roots are sliced into sections measuring about ¾ inches (2 cm) thick and parboiled. The root pieces are then placed on screens in the sun to dry, being covered at night to keep off the dew, and turned occasionally to promote even drying. When the pieces are thoroughly dry, they may be stored for later use, ground up, and used as "unprocessed root," or they may be further processed according to the "black bean" method. In short, this method involves long simmering of the dried root pieces in the gravy leftover from cooking black beans.

Tincture of dried, cured or uncured root: 1:5 (50A:50W)

Water extract: Basic decoction of dried, cured or uncured root.

Practical uses (uncured root): Eliminative tonic for treating bad skin, constipation, and high blood cholesterol.

Practical uses (cured root): This is one of the most respected tonic herbs of TCM. He-shou-wu is an energy and sexual tonic. The herb improves the function of liver and kidneys, builds blood, and promotes longevity.

Dosage: According to basic recommendations found under "Dosage of tinctures," pages 49–52 and "Dosage of teas and decoctions," pages 70–71.

Contraindications: The uncured root has a laxative effect that may be accompanied by unpleasant griping sensations. The slow cooking of the cured root is designed to lessen this effect.

Hops (*Humulus lupulus*)
Family: Hemp (*Cannabaceae*)

Part used: The lupulin-rich strobiles (the bright-green, conelike female flower) used fresh or recently dried. The strobile is best picked at peak ripeness, when the dustlike, yellow lupulin is richly apparent and before the scales that comprise the strobile show any signs of browning at the edges. Since the resins and essential oils present in the lupulin are apt to degrade and volatilize during storage, it is best to use the strobile (the hops) soon after harvest. Dried hops may be kept reasonably fresh for up to 6 months, packed tightly in an airtight container and refrigerated. Different hops cultivars are characterized by their taste and aroma, as well as on the basis of "alpha." Alpha refers to the percentage of total alpha acids (composed mainly of the molecule humulone) compared to the total dry weight. Various cultivars will range from alpha 4 to alpha 19, with alpha 4 being mildly bitter, and alpha 19 being extremely bitter. The higher the alpha, the stronger the medicine.

Tincture of fresh hops: 1:2 (100A) Use Blender method (p. 22).

Tincture of dry hops: 1:5 (65A:35W)

Folk method for preparing hops tincture: Pack the fresh strobiles tightly in a jar and cover with grain alcohol or unflavored vodka. Macerate with daily shaking for 2 weeks, then squeeze through a cheesecloth, or use the tincture press. This method makes a more dilute tincture, preserves more of the delicate aroma of the hops, and is a bit less overpowering than the standard tinctures that are made from ground-up strobiles.

Water extracts: Tea made by combining 2 teaspoons of dried hops in 1 cup of boiling water. Allow to steep for 4 minutes before straining and drinking.

Beer: The value of hops in beer manufacture is multifaceted, including: bittering, flavoring, imparting aroma, and preservation. Hops stobiles are added during the boiling of the wort, usually in 3 phases. The first addition is timed to the beginning of boiling, allowing for extraction of the resinous *bitter* agent. Bitterness is necessary in beer, in order to counteract the syrupy sweetness of the malt. The second addition of hops is usually made when there are only about 15 minutes remaining to the boil, in order to impart a crisp hop *flavor* to the beer. The third addition is made after the brew kettle has been removed from the fire, or (in the case of dry hopping) during the fermentation process. This late addition of hops captures the volatile oils, which are responsible for the *aroma* of the beer. Regardless of when it is added, hops has a preservative effect on the beer by discouraging the growth of yeasts and gram positive bacteria. The hops disarms these organisms, thereby extending the shelf-life of the beer.

Practical uses: The tea and tincture may be taken for the mild narcotic action. Irritation, muscle tightness, nervousness, tension headache, menstrual cramping, and insomnia all yield to the relaxing, sedative, and analgesic effects of the yellow-dusted hops strobile. Hops is also effective in treating premature ejaculation in males. The medicinal effects are probably best achieved by using hops in the form of tea or tincture. Used in the form of beer, some of the positive attributes may be counteracted: The mellow mood may give way to the pugilism of the drinker, or the long-lasting erection may be softened by the alcohol.

Dosage: According to basic recommendations found under "Dosage of tinctures," pages 49–52.

Contraindications and cautions: Anyone who has picked hops knows that one really needs to reach into the plant to get the goods, and that the vine itself is very rough, which causes irritated scratches on the hands and arms. Pick early in the day, and wear protective apparel! Hops is mildly proestrogenic. While moderate use is not a problem, habitual use may increase estrogen, which can be a contributing factor to breast cancer. Therefore, women taking this herb to relax, or to relieve menstrual pain, are advised to use only as needed, not on a long-term basis. Men using hops on a daily basis may develop "beer breasts," and sex drive may diminish. Finally, hops therapy is not recommended for those suffering from deep depression, as the sedative effects can potentiate despondence.

Horehound (*Marrubium vulgare*)
Family: Mint (*Lamiaceae*)

Part used: Leaf and flower, harvested in early flowering stage and used fresh or dried.

Tincture of fresh herb: 1:2 (75A:25W)

Tincture of dry herb: 1:5 (50A:50W)

Water extracts: Basic tea or decoction of fresh or dried herb.

Cough syrup: 1 part by volume of a strong decoction of the fresh herb is combined with 2 parts by volume of honey (see "Chapter 9, Herbal Succi and Syrups," pages 76–9).

Soft extract: Make a strong decoction and simmer slowly in a saucepan, while stirring contantly. The solution will thicken into the soft extract, which may be dried into lozenges. See page 70.

Practical uses: Horehound soothes the upper respiratory tract, suppresses coughing, and promotes expectoration. The gentle laxative and digestive bitter effects are also helpful for treating the common cold, which is a condition of congestion and bodily stasis. Horehound gets things moving. Taken as a hot tea, the herb will help bring on delayed menstruation.

Dosage: According to basic recommendations found under "Dosage of tinctures," pages 49–52 and "Dosage of teas and decoctions," pages 70–71.

Contraindications: Do not take large amounts during pregnancy.

Horse Chestnut (Conker Tree)
(*Aesculus hippocastanum*)
Family: Soapberry (*Sapindaceae*)

Parts used: The fresh or dried leaf, bark of twig, bark of root, resiny buds, and most importantly the fruit (the seed, the nut, the conker). The seed contains the highest concentration of active constituents, the mixture of saponins collectively known as aescin. The resiny buds and bark are best harvested in the early spring, as the sap begins to rise, but before the tree leafs out. The leaf may be harvested any time during the growing season. The mahogany-brown nuts are harvested after the spiked pericarp splits, and are air-dried (whole) for at least 2 days before grinding and extracting. This lessens the water content of the seed, which helps to standardize the tincture and keeps the oil infusion from rotting during extraction.

Tincture of seed: 1:5 (60A:40W). Chop, cut, or snip the nuts into pieces and use the blender method (see page 22).

Oil, salve, or cream: Make infused herbal oil of fresh or dried leaf, bark, or bud, using the formulas found in "Chapter 10, Basic Formulas for Herbal Oils, Salves, and Creams," pages 85–86. This oil can be used as-is or may be further processed into salve or cream. Making herbal oil out of conkers (horse chestnut seeds) requires less time, a higher heat, and a different formula. Cut or snip the nuts into pieces, then pulverize coarsely in a blender or by running at loose setting through a grain mill. Use the seed coat as well as the fatty portions of the seed. The formula is 1:3 (100% oil). Heat to 150° F (65° C), stirring at least 3 times a day, for 2 days (48 hours), then press, settle, decant, filter, and bottle in the usual manner. This oil can be used as-is or may be further processed into salve or cream (see pages 87–90).

Practical uses: Horse chestnut helps tonify the circulatory system. Taken internally in the form of the tincture, or applied externally as an oily preparation, the herb helps shrink boggy veins, tightening their walls and rendering them more elastic. This stimulates blood flow from the lower extremities back up to the heart. Horse chestnut helps prevent coagulation or clotting

197

(thrombus) of the blood inside circulatory system, and reduces inflammation of the veins (phlebitis). The herb reduces edema (fluid retention) by increasing the permeability of the capillaries, allowing the reabsorption and healthy redistribution of liquids once held in boggy tissues. Herbal preparations of horse chestnut are used for treating varicose veins, leg ulcers, tired legs, painful legs, swollen lower legs and ankles, sports injuries, muscle cramps and hemorrhoids.

Dosage: 2 to 4 drops up to 3 times per day, diluted in a whole glass of water and/or with food. This is a low dose botanical. The oil, salve or cream may be safely applied to the affected areas as often and as liberally as needed.

Contraindications:

Internal: Take the tincture only at the recommendation of a qualified health care practitioner. Do not use in conjunction with coumadin, warfarin, or aspirin, as the blood thinning properties of these medications may be potentiated by horse chestnut. Do not use if suffering from liver or kidney disease. Discontinue use if symptoms of nausea or headache occur.

External: External use in rare cases may cause a rash, in which case discontinue use.

Horseradish (*Cochlearia armoracea*)
Family: *Mustard* (*Brassicaceae*)

Parts used: The fresh or dried root.

Tincture of dried root: 1:5 (50A:50W) Grind the dried root to a powder, weigh it, and pour into a macerating vessel. Then, add the water part of the menstruum only, stirring to moisten the herb. Allow to sit overnight in the closed vessel (giving time for an enzymatic reaction to occur, maximizing the production of medicinally active allyl mustard oil). In the morning, add the alcohol portion of the menstruum. This arrests all enzymatic activity. Shake well, then macerate, press, and filter as usual. Horseradish tincture acts to open the sinus passages and serves as a potent vascular stimulant, warming the extremities and accelerating the healing process. Used alone or combined with complimentary tinctures, this preparation is useful for treating upper respiratory disorders—sinus infection and the common cold; also treats urinary tract infection, atonic digestion, rheumatism, and gout.

Dosage: According to basic recommendations found under "Dosage of tinctures," pages 49–52.

Syrup: In a well-ventilated room, grate fresh horseradish root into a bowl and allow to sit for at least 3 minutes. This gives time for the enzymatic reaction to occur, maximizing the pungency and, therefore, the medicinality of the syrup. Then, transfer the root into a canning jar (use a spoon) and add sufficient raw honey to cover. Allow to sit at room temperature for 30 days, then press through cheesecloth. Store the finished syrup in a stoppered bottle, out of the light. Take in tablespoonful doses as needed for treating sinusitis, sinus headache, allergies, hoarseness, or cough.

Condiment: In a well-ventilated room, finely grate fresh horseradish root into a bowl and allow to sit for at least 3 minutes. This gives time for the enzymatic reaction to occur, maximizing the pungency and, therefore, the medicinality of the sauce. For each cup of grated horseradish, add 3 tablespoonsful of apple cider vinegar and ½ teaspoon of salt. Mix thoroughly, then store in a lidded jar in the refrigerator. The sauce is ready to use immediately and will last up to 3 months without undue deterioration. Use as desired for dressing rich foods, meats, and on sandwiches. This condiment stimulates the gastric secretions and warms the digestive fire, while protecting against bacterial pathogens, including *Staphylococcus aureus* and *Escherichia coli.*

Direct consumption: 1 teaspoonful of freshly grated root taken before meals or as needed, with honey—only if you dare.

Contraindications: Discontinue use if the horseradish causes gastrointestinal discomfort. Not to be used by those suffering from stomach or intestinal ulcers.

Hyssop (*Hyssopus officinalis*)
Family: Mint (*Lamiaceae*)

Parts used: Leaf and flower (without the stems) harvested at the peak of flowering and used fresh or dried. Harvest carefully to avoid bruising the herb, which is easily discolored and may lose volatile oils during handling. Spread thinly on screens or hang in sparse bundles in the shade. Careful turning, good air flow, and low heat will help conserve the delicate aroma of the herb. Once the branches are quite dry, working over a clean table, hand-strip the leaves and flowers from the stem, keeping them in a neat pile. Store the leaf and flower in a glass jar, and rub or grind them just prior to making the tincture or tea.

Tincture of fresh herb: 1:2 (100A); see page 37.

Tincture of dried herb: 1:5 (75A:25W)

Water extract: Basic tea of fresh or dried herb.

Cough syrup: Combine 1 part by volume of a strong tea of the dried herb with 2 parts by volume of honey. Delicious! See "Chapter 9, Herbal Succi and Syrups," pages 77–78.

Sunny honey: Pack a crock or jar with fresh flowering tops and cover in honey, allowing to steep for 2 weeks on a sunny windowsill. Then, press out over a bowl, using a cheesecloth, or press out in a tincture press. Discard the marc and bottle the honey. This may be taken by the teaspoonful as often as needed, to allay sore throat, cough, tonsillitis, and/or laryngitis.

Practical uses: Hyssop is a stimulating expectorant demonstrating marked antiviral activity. The herb promotes elimination of toxins via sweating and diuretic effects. The specific application is in symptomatic relief and swift resolution of the common cold.

Dosage: According to basic recommendations found under "Dosage of tinctures," pages 49–52 and "Dosage of teas and decoctions," pages 70–71.

Contraindications: Not to be used during pregnancy. Avoid direct contact with pure, undiluted essential oil of hyssop, especially on sensitive skin, mucous membranes, and in eyes.

$\mathcal{J}$

Indigo, Wild (*Baptisia tinctoria*)
Family: Legume (*Fabaceae*)

Parts used: Root harvested during dormancy and used fresh or dried. Wash roots thoroughly in cold water. Leaves harvested just prior to flowering and used fresh or dried.

Tincture of fresh root (preferred): 1:2 (75A:25W)

Tincture of dried root: 1:5 (50A:50W)

Water extracts: Basic tea of fresh or dried leaves (for external use only). Basic decoction of fresh or dried root.

Practical uses: Wild indigo is best used for treating recurring infections of the mucous membranes of the mouth and throat typified by purplish coloration and fullness of tissue, including mouth sores, tumors, spongy gums, sore throat, and tonsillitis. It is antiseptic, mildly astringent, and stimulating to the lymph, liver, and bowels. Wild indigo works locally against infection, improving the tone of the tissues, while stimulating expulsion of toxic metabolic waste. For this purpose, the herb combines well with cleavers. The use of wild indigo in treating wasting diseases, cellular degeneration, and cancer should not be overlooked.

Dosage: Starting adult dosage is 1 dropperful of the tincture (30 drops) diluted in 1 cup of water (240 ml) taken 3 to 5 times daily. The dosage of the decoction is ½ cup (120 ml) taken 2 to 3 times daily. The course of treatment should not be extended beyond the time required to resolve the problem. See "Contraindications."

External: The diluted tincture can be taken internally and used simultaneously as a gargle. The tea of the leaves or the root decoction can be used as a wash or compress for treating slow-to-heal ulcerations of the skin or mucous membranes, applied several times during the day, and the area left open to the air between applications. The tincture can be used in the same manner, 2 droppersful (60 drops) diluted in 1 cup (240 ml) of cold water.

Oil, salve, or cream: Make infused herbal oil of the fresh or dried leaves. This may be used as-is or as an ingredient for making salve or cream according to the procedure found in "Chapter 10, Basic Formulas for Herbal Oils, Salves, and Creams." The oily extracts may be applied externally to swollen lymph nodes, mastitis, tumors, or slow-healing ulcerations.

Contraindications: Not to be taken during pregnancy. Wild indigo is strong medicine and should be used under the care of a qualified health professional. Do not exceed recommended dosage. Overdose can cause violent purging. Leaves are for making the water extract for external use only.

Other species: "False indigo" (*Baptisia australis*), which is indigenous to North America, is often used as a substitute for wild indigo (*Baptisia tinctoria*). Several other strains of indigo were introduced into the New World as dye plants by early settlers in times predating the Louisiana purchase, and these have escaped into the wild. Wild indigo may be readily identified by the bright yellow flowers that give way to characteristic blue-black seedpods, pointed at the tip and about the size of a pea. In order to address the problem of diminishing supplies of wild-harvested wild indigo, and to assure the identity of the herb in commerce, responsible cultivation of correctly identified *B. tinctoria* is a very high priority. This can best be accomplished by growers in coastal areas of the south, where the winters are mild, the summers are humid, and the soil is sandy. By the way, so-called "true indigo," (*Indigofera tinctoria*) is from a different genus and is not a substitute for wild indigo.

$\mathcal{J}$

Jewelweed (*Impatiens capensis, I. pallida*)
Family: Balsam (*Balsaminaceae*)

Parts used: The entire fresh flowering plant, including the root, picked in the early morning (when bejewelled by dew) and processed immediately. Roots should be kept attached to the plant, trimmed of rootlets, and thoroughly washed to remove remaining dirt particles. Store whole plants in wet sheets for transport.

Tincture of fresh herb: 1:2 (100A) Blender method (p. 22). For external use only (see "Contraindications").

Tincturing with witch hazel: 1:2 (100 witch hazel extract) Blender method, but instead of using alcohol, use witch hazel extract (14% alcohol), a common remedy that can be purchased at any drugstore. Jewelweed tincture made using witch hazel extract has a 1-year shelf-life and must be kept refrigerated. The powerful astringency of witch hazel compliments the anti-inflammatory activity of the jewelweed.

Succus of fresh whole plant: 1 part alcohol by vol.:3 parts jewelweed juice by vol. (see "Chapter 9, Herbal Succi and Syrups," pages 73–75). Take care to add the alcohol incrementally during pressing, in order to preserve the juice from degradation, which can be rapid. The juice will turn dark green or red upon addition of alcohol, which is indicative of the presence of the antihistamine and anti-inflammatory molecule known as lawsone (hennatonic acid). Lawsone is also present in the tincture, the fresh juice, and the water extract.

Water extract: Pack whole, fresh herb tightly in a stainless steel saucepan and cover with water. Simmer on low heat for 15 minutes, strain to remove plant material, then return the liquid to the saucepan and reduce on low heat to 50% volume. Cool to room temperature and use immediately, refrigerate in clean glass for up to a week, or freeze in ice cube trays for prolonged (frozen) storage. Jewelweed ice cubes on beesting—aahh!

Poultice or wash: Mash the fresh plant by folding and worrying until the juices flow, then apply as a poultice, or simply rub the juice on the affected area. The poultice or wash may be made of aerial parts without the roots. Younger plants (pre-flowering) work just as well as the mature plant.

Oil, salve, or cream: Make infused herbal oil of the fresh plant. Jewelweed is indeed oil-soluble, but its tissues are delicate and watery—easily extracted in oil, yet likely to ferment during extraction. Here are some suggestions: Allow the herb to wilt overnight prior to extraction. Chop the fresh herb coarsely in order to limit juiciness. Make sure the mass is completely covered by oil in the cooker. Stir to release air bubbles. Digest for 2 days only, not 1 week. If the oil starts to ferment (visible as active bubbling of the ingredients), raise the temperature to 150° F (65° C). Stir constantly until all bubbling ceases. Then, cool the mixture back down, press out the oil, settle overnight, and decant without further delay. Once the oil has been rendered free of water, it will store reasonably well, and may be used as-is or may be further processed into salve or cream. Personally, I prefer the fresh juice or the alcoholic preparations in treatment of poison oak and ivy, because I find that the emolliency of the oil tends to exacerbate the inflammation, but some people swear by it. The oily preparations are good for treating old burns and hemorrhoids. See "Chapter 10, Basic Formulas for Herbal Oils, Salves, and Creams," page 83, also pages 87–90.

Practical uses: The fresh plant poultice of jewelweed is the best spontaneous trailside remedy for preventing and treating poison oak or ivy rash. As a prophylactic, the juice may be rubbed on prior to exposure. Jewelweed prohibits adsorption of urushiol (the resin in poison oak and ivy that causes so much suffering among the naked ape clan). This is not to dissuade poison ivy sufferers from washing the skin and clothing after exposure—this, too, is an excellent practice. Jewelweed, when applied to existing poison oak or ivy rash, has a strong antihistamine effect, reducing on-site inflammation, preventing weeping, spread, and tissue damage. The herb reduces itching and promotes rapid healing. Jewelweed may also be useful for treating other histamine-related inflammations, including mosquito bites, beestings, nettle stings, and hives.

Contraindications: External use only. This plant is not recommended for internal use, due to the high oxalic acid and selenium content. The poultice and water extracts are safe for external application. The tincture and the succus are generally well-tolerated, although adverse reactions have been reported. These products should inhibit (not potentiate!) inflammation. A small patch test may be performed prior to wholesale application. If adverse reactions occur, do not use.

Other species: Chinese balsam (*Impatiens balsamina*) contains a watery mucilage similar to that provided by our American species. Chinese balsam also contains the molecule lawsone, and may be used interchangeably with jewelweed.

Jiao-gu-lan (Immortality, Amachazuru)
(*Gynostemma pentaphyllum*)
Family: Gourd (*Cucurbitaceae*)

Parts used: The leaves and succulent stems of the vine, used fresh or dried.

Tincture of fresh herb: 1:2 (50A:50W)

Tincture of dried herb: 1:5 (25A:75W)
Active constituents of jiao-gu-lan (saponins and polysaccharides) are fully water-soluble. The fresh herb has a complex taste— sweetish at first and then bitter. The tinctures have a similar taste, whether made from fresh or dry herb.

Glycerite of fresh herb: 1:2 (100Gly)

Water extract: Basic tea of dried herb. This is the traditional and recommended way to take jiao-gu-lan. Drying the leaves and making them into tea augments the sweeter taste of the herb and subdues the bitterness, while delivering the health-promoting aspects in the most agreeable form. The tea tastes very much like tea of nettles.

205

Direct consumption: Eat 1 or 2 fresh leaves daily.

Practical uses: Although jiao-gu-lan is only a recent introduction to the Chinese pharmacopoeia, there has been a longstanding folk tradition of using the herb. For centuries, inhabitants of the mountains of southern China and rural communities of Japan have brewed the tea to promote general well-being and long life. Since the early 1970s, research groups have worked diligently to identify the active constituents and test the activity of the herb. The agents responsible for the noteworthy effects are saponins classed as "gypenosides," very similar in their chemical makeup to the ginsenosides found in ginseng and present in surprisingly high concentrations. Jiao-gu-lan demonstrates strong adaptogenic activity, increasing athletic endurance while reducing the negative effects of stress—both physical and emotional. Taken on an ongoing basis, the herb demonstrates a normalizing effect on blood pressure, depending on the needs of the individual (low blood pressure is raised to normal levels or, conversely, high blood pressure is lowered to safe levels). In fact, many of the benefits of the herb may be traced to its positive influence on the vascular system, circulation, and cells of the blood. There is a profound antioxidant effect, with a lowering of free radical damage. Jiao-gu-lan improves circulation by reducing fatty sedimentation in the blood vessels. In conjunction with exercise, this herb quickens fat metabolism and has been used effectively in weight loss programs. Much like garlic, jiao-gu-lan lessens blood platelet aggregation, providing significant protection from stroke or heart attack, even in predisposed individuals. The immuno-stimulating activity revolves around increased production of white blood cells, especially in immune-depressed individuals and those who have recently undergone radiation or chemotherapy. Daily use of the tea may be expected to significantly speed recovery from debilitating illness. Positive results have also been recorded in the areas of cancer prevention and the shrinking of tumors. Finally, the herb shows promise in treating both hepatitis B and diabetes.

Dosage: According to basic recommendations found under "Dosage of tinctures," pages 49–52, "Dosage of glycerites," page 63, and "Dosage of teas and decoctions," pages 70–71. The tea has a positive tonic effect when taken once daily over a period of several weeks. More vigorous therapy (including athletic training, weight loss, and treatment of overt disease states) may require an increased dosage—up to 3 cups of tea daily.

Contraindications: Due to the effects on blood platelet aggregation, jiao-gu-lan should not be taken in conjunction with the pharmaceutical anticoagulant warfarin. Otherwise, the herb is safe when administered at the recommended dosage.

Ju-hua (*Chrysanthemum morifolium*)
Family: Aster (*Asteraceae*)

Parts used: Entire flowers, picked during early maturity, laid out on screens in the shade, and turned frequently until dry. Remove all stems and leaves. Store the lightweight, fluffy, pleasantly aromatic flowers whole, in a sealed container, in the refrigerator.

Tincture of dried flowers: 1:5 (50A:50W)

Tea of dried flowers: 1:30 (use 50 g dried flowers and 1500 ml water). Place flowers in the teapot, cover with boiling water and allow to steep for 4 minutes, then pour off through a strainer. Sometimes the tea is made in a saucepan and the flowers are briefly simmered (10 minutes) prior to steeping. Moist flowers in the bottom of the teapot may be brewed once again by adding more hot water. This is often done up to 3 times.

Medicated wine (*Vina medicata*): Use white wine from grapes (9 to 16% alcohol content) or Chinese rice wine (18 to 25% alcohol). Place 100 g of whole ju-hua flowers in a glass jar and add 1000 ml of wine. Close tightly and macerate in a warm, dark place for 7 to 10 days, with daily shaking. At this time, pour off the wine through a strainer or cheesecloth, discard the flowers and keep the medicated wine in a new container, well-stoppered. Dosage is ½ wineglassful once or twice daily. In China, this is known as "auspicious wine" and is traditionally imbibed during the Double Ninth Festival. This practice is said to divert disaster and bring good fortune. Used medicinally, the wine soothes the stomach, replenishes vital force, helps reduce blood pressure, and promotes healthy circulation of the blood.

Practical uses: Ju-hua is one of the main Chinese herbs that releases the exterior, used in the form of tea or tincture for treating common colds, flu, fever, and heatstroke; high blood pressure, heart pain (angina), atherosclerosis; dizziness, hearing loss, tinnitus, headache and migraine; red and swollen eyes, blurry vision; liver inflammation and toxicity; infections including staphylococcus, streptococcus, and blood spirochetes. The herb has a cooling and detoxifying effect for treating these acute conditions, but is also commonly used in the form of a daily tisane, a tonic to promote energy, improve hearing and vision, stimulate intelligence and mental acuity, and promote longevity.

Yellow Chrysanthemum flower (huang-ju-hua) is larger in size, somewhat bitter to the taste and cooling. The yellow color is indicative of lutein content, making it a specific for treating eye disease, including age-related macular degeneration.

White Chrysanthemum flower (bai-ju-hua) is smaller in size, smelling antiseptic, and somewhat sweeter to the taste. The herb calms the liver and benefits the eyes.

Autumn-flowering Chrysanthemum (*Huangshan-gongzhu*) bears small flowers with bright yellow centers and creamy ray flowers. This variety hails from the Yellow Mountains in Eastern China. In the year 2010, we received cuttings of this cultivar and introduced it successfully to our gardens. The bushes become studded with flowers very late in the season, softened and made sweeter by the influence of frosty nights. Propagation is by crown division or cuttings only. Like the other domesticated *Chrysanthemum* cultivars, the plant long ago lost its ability to reproduce from seed.

Dosage: Tincture: As a daily tonic, take 10 to 30 drops of the tincture before meals. For acute symptoms, take 20 to 40 drops up to 5 times a day. Tea: As a daily tonic, take 1 cup of tea up to 3 times a day, before meals. For treating acute symptoms, make the tea very strong by simmering for 10 minutes, and take as often as needed until the problem is resolved.

Contraindications: The herb is considered safe for general consumption, although rare cases of allergic reaction to this and other members of the Aster family can occur. Due to the presence of sesquiterpene lactones, sensitive individuals may experience contact dermatitis during harvest—wear gloves, and keep hands that are covered with plant juices out of eyes. Wash well after handling.

Other species: *Chrysanthemum indicum* (ye-ju-hua) is the wild counterpart to the mildly-flavored cultivars that are more commonly used to make chrysanthemum tea. Ye-ju-hua is considered one of the Chinese herbs that clears heat, being very powerful in its action. The herb may be taken as a tea and is also commonly used as a fresh plant poultice (entire plant, mashed) to treat boils and abscesses.

Juniper (*Juniperus communis*)
Family: Cypress (*Cupressaceae*)

Parts used: The ripe female cones (the berries) harvested in the fall when they turn purple, then gently shade-dried. The roots, leaves, branches, gum, bark, and wood of juniper are also employed extensively in traditional (especially Native American) herbal medicine. Historically, both the Okanagan Indians and the Potawatomi used juniper berries in the same way modern herbalists use them—to treat urinary tract infection.

Tincture of dried berry: 1:4 (90A:10W) Soak the whole berries in the menstruum overnight, then in the morning blend them up and pour into a macerating container. Macerate, press, settle, and filter according to the standard procedures. Store in amber glass. To clean up, a clean rag dipped in pure grain alcohol will help dissolve the resins that coat every surface of blender and press.

Water extract: Basic tea made by pouring 1 cup of hot water over ½ teaspoon of dried, crushed juniper berries and 1 teaspoon dried licorice root. Allow to steep 5 to 10 minutes, strain, and drink.

Practical uses: The tincture or tea of juniper berries is one of the best of all urinary tract antiseptics. It is commonly used in tea blends or compound tinctures, combined at a rate of 1 part in 10, with the juniper berries making up the smaller part of the formula. The greater part of the formula would consist of one or more demulcent and diuretic herbs combined, such as: corn silk, goldenrod, licorice, linden, marshmallow, slippery elm, or uva ursi. This formula makes one of the best treatments for subacute or chronic urinary tract infection or inflammation of the kidneys, bladder and/or urethra. These conditions are characterized by symptoms such as frequent urination, burning urine, a feeling of incomplete urinary discharge, pain or itching in the urinary tract.

Dosage: As previously mentioned, this herb is best used in formula at a concentration of 1:10. If using Juniper berries alone, take the tea (up to 3 cups daily) at the first signs of urinary discomfort. Take the tincture at the rate of 3 to 5 drops, up to 3 times a day, well-diluted in water. See UTI formula below.

Contraindications: Not to be used during menstruation, pregnancy, or in the presence of kidney disease. Large doses, unless accompanied by a demulcent, can irritate the urinary passages and may cause gastric distress.

* * * * * * *

UTI Formula: Mix together 5 parts goldenrod tincture, 4 parts marshmallow tincture, and 1 part tincture of juniper berries. Take 30 drops in a cup of water 3 to 5 times daily or as needed to allay symptoms of urinary tract infection. Avoid refined carbohydrates and processed sugar.

Khella (*Ammi visnaga*)
Family: Carrot (*Apiaceae*)

Part used: Seed harvested at maturity and dried.

Tincture of seed: 1:4 (75A:25W)
The seeds can be ground up or bruised, soaked overnight in the menstruum, then briefly blended the following day and macerated in the usual manner.

Practical uses: Khella is an efficient and nonstimulating bronchial dilator used in treating asthma and emphysema. It is not very effective to use during emergency asthma attacks, but rather is taken on an ongoing basis as a preventive. The herb is a serviceable antispasmodic for assisting in the passing of stones from the urinary tract. Due to its vasodilating effects, it is also used to treat arteriosclerosis. Combine with garlic or jiao-gu-lan.

Dosage: According to basic recommendations found under "Dosage of tinctures," pages 49–52.

Contraindications: Rare allergic reactions have been recorded, but overall the herb is well-tolerated and nontoxic. However, internal use of khella can cause skin photosensitivity. During the course of treatment, long exposure to the sun should be avoided. Do not exceed recommended dosage.

Other species: Bishop's weed (*Ammi majus*) is a close botanical relative, but the herb is not used interchangeably with khella for the bronchial dilating, antispasmodic, or vasodilating effects. Instead, bishop's weed seed has come under investigation for treating vitiligo (piebald skin). The herb is taken internally and the liquid extract is also painted on the skin. Over time, and after periodic exposure to the sun, this therapy often results in restoration of pigmentation. Given the photosensitizing effects of khella, it may prove that both khella and bishop's weed can be used interchangeably for treating vitiligo.

Lady's Mantle (*Alchemilla vulgaris*)
Family: Rose (*Rosaceae*)

Parts used: Entire aerial parts, including leaves, flowers, and stems, harvested in the early flowering stage and used fresh or dried. When making the fresh extract, it is good to harvest before the sun evaporates the glistening and magnifying dewdrops from the leaves, since these unique orbs are considered to carry great virtue. The fresh or dried root is medicinally interchangeable with the aerial parts, but the aerial parts are nonetheless preferred, since digging the root kills the plant.

Tincture of fresh herb: 1:2 (75A:15W:10Gly)

Tincture of dried herb: 1:5 (50A:40W:10Gly)
Glycerin is added to the tinctures in order to stabilize the tannins, which are the main active constituents in lady's mantle. This produces an elegant preparation.

Glycerite of fresh herb: 1:2 (100Gly)

Water extract: Basic tea of dried herb.

Practical uses: As its name implies, lady's mantle is an herb dedicated to women and may be used with good effect to invigorate and tonify the female sexual organs. For treating excessive menstrual bleeding or leukorrhea, the tea, tincture, or glycerite may be taken internally and the cooled tea or diluted tincture used concurrently as a douche. As a harmless pregnancy tonic, the herb helps allay morning sickness, assists in easy childbirth, and encourages rapid postpartum recuperation. Subtly bolstering the mind, lady's mantle may be of assistance in amending grief over miscarriage, postpartum depression, or the mood swings of menopause.

Dosage: According to basic recommendations found under "Dosage of tinctures," pages 49–52, "Dosage of glycerites," page 63, and "Dosage of teas and decoctions," pages 70–71.

Contraindications: None known. Safe for general use.

Lavender
(*Lavandula* spp.)
Family: Mint (*Lamiaceae*)

Part used: Flowering heads harvested in the early flowering stage and used fresh or dried.

Tincture of fresh flowers: 1:2 (100A)

Tincture of dried flowers: 1:5 (75A:25W)

Water extract: Basic tea of dried flowering heads.

Practical uses: Lavender is a mild sedative for treating headache, nervousness, and nervous insomnia. Simply smelling the living flowers or a bundle of the dried flowering stalks is an uplifting experience, especially good for convalescents. Lavender is also a digestive remedy, especially useful for treating any sensation of overfullness or nausea after eating.

Dosage: According to basic recommendations found under "Dosage of tinctures," pages 49–52 and "Dosage of teas and decoctions," pages 70–71.

Food use: Cookies made with lavender flowers as an ingredient are, quite frankly, awful.

External: The tincture may be rubbed full-strength on the temples to treat headache and insomnia. To discourage lice infestation, apply the essential oil or the tincture directly to the hair or to the hairbrush. To speed the healing of burns, open sores, or infections, prepare a compress or wash with the cold tea or the tincture diluted at the rate of 2 droppersful (60 drops) per cup (240 ml) of distilled water. Allow the area to dry in the air between applications. The lavender bath is prepared by putting several handfuls of lavender in a muslin bag (basically a giant tea bag) and tying it shut with string, then running hot bath water over it. Such a bath is sedative to the nerves.

Contraindications: Safe for general use. However, the pure essential oil of lavender is best kept out of the eyes and away from sensitive mucous membranes.

Other species: The open-pollinated lavenders, consisting of true English lavender (*Lavandula angustifolia vera*), broadleaf lavender (*L. latifolia*), and French lavender (*L. stoechas*) have distinct aromas, but can be used interchangeably in medicine. The popular cultivars of English lavender (e.g. hidcote and munstead lavenders) are also used interchangeably for medicine. Hybrid lavenders (*L. angustifolia x L. latifolia*) consisting of the several named varieties (e.g. *delphinensis, grosso, provence*) are also used medicinally, yielding a high volume of low-grade essential oil. The open-pollinated lavenders yield higher-grade essential oils.

Lemon Balm (*Melissa officinalis*)
Family: Mint (*Lamiaceae*)

Parts used: Leaf and flower, without the stems, harvested in the early flowering stage and used fresh or dried.

Tincture of fresh herb: 1:2 (100A)

Tincture of dried herb: 1:5 (75A:25W)

Water extract: Basic tea of fresh or dried herb.

Juice or succus: The fresh leaves may be juiced and taken straight. To make a preserved lemon balm succus, add 1 part by volume of grain alcohol to 3 parts by volume of fresh juice (see "Chapter 9, Herbal Succi and Syrups," pages 73–5).

Practical uses: Lemon balm promotes longevity. It is a gently sedative and calming herb, especially useful for treating nervousness of adults and overexcitement of children. For treating the common cold, the herb has a mild antiviral influence and helps sweat out a fever. Daily consumption of the fresh juice or succus may assist in regulating hyperactive thyroid—potentially helpful in treating goiter and Grave's disease. Lemon balm improves the taste and activity of other herbs. When used in combination with laxatives, it has a complimentary antispasmodic effect.

Dosage: According to basic recommendations found under "Dosage of tinctures," pages 49–52 and "Dosage of teas and decoctions," pages 70–71.

External: The tincture or tea is specific for herpes and may be applied full strength to the lesions; for this purpose, combines well with self-heal.

Contraindications: None known. Safe for general use.

Licorice (*Glycyrrhiza glabra, G. uralensis*) Family: Legume (*Fabaceae*)

Parts used: The root dug during dormancy, after 3 years of growth, and used fresh or dried. Root harvested in the spring, just before the growth phase, is of highest quality.

Tincture: The basic methods for making a tincture do not apply to licorice, because soaking the ground root in an alcoholic menstruum leads to the extraction of bitter tannins and results in a very inferior extract. As with astragalus, the best mode of preparation is to make a strong decoction and preserve by adding sufficient grain alcohol to bring the final absolute alcohol content to 20%.

Water extracts (preferred): Basic tea or decoction of the sliced, fresh or dried root.

Direct consumption: "Licorice sticks" consist of fresh or dried sections of licorice root. These can be chewed as needed, and are often used in treating tobacco addiction, providing a tactile substitute to cigarettes and also facilitating discharge of mucous from the upper respiratory tract.

Practical uses: Licorice supports adrenal function. It is a useful demulcent and anti-inflammatory for treating irritated mucous membranes and stomach or duodenal ulcer, also stimulating repair and regeneration of these tissues. Licorice is commonly used in herbal formulas, as a flavoring agent and to harmonize and enhance the activities of other herbs.

Dosage: According to basic recommendations found under "Dosage of tinctures," pages 49–52 and "Dosage of teas and decoctions," pages 70–71. Do not exceed recommended dosage. Liquid extracts of licorice are incompatible with acids and should not be taken in citric juices.

Contraindications: Not to be used during pregnancy or nursing. Large doses or excessive long-term usage (exceeding 4 to 6 weeks) may cause potassium depletion and sodium retention, which is undesirable. This can, in turn, cause increased sensitivity to heart medicines containing cardiac glycosides. A diet that includes apple cider vinegar, bananas, and dried apricots can be followed while using licorice, in order to bolster potassium levels. Use of licorice is contraindicated for diabetics and those suffering from hypertension.

Other species: Several other species of *Glycyrrhiza* are used locally in China and Eastern Europe as substitutes for true licorice. These include *G. korshinskyi*, *G. yunnanensis*, and *G. echinata*. Wild American licorice (*G. lepidota*), is native to the American Rocky Mountains and is sometimes used by locals as a substitute for true licorice. It is not sweet and is far inferior in its effect.

Linden (Little-leaf Lime) (*Tilia cordata*)
Family: Mallow (*Malvaceae*)

Parts used: The main medicine consists of the flower cluster and bract. Flowers are aromatic and creamy-white, subtending the light-green, skateboard-like bract. The flower cluster and bract are picked together at early maturity and promptly dried. This product is highly susceptible to damage from moisture and sunlight. Store in whole form, in sealed containers in the refrigerator. Linden leaves, bark, and the wood of the tree are also usefully employed in medicinal context. Leaves may be used fresh or dried, while the bark and the wood may be slow-burned in a low oxygen environment to produce adsorptive charcoal (carbon).

Tincture of dried flower and bract: 1:4 (50A:30W:20GLY) Grind the herb and weigh it, mix the menstruum according to formula, pour over the dried herb, and stopper immediately and shake to incorporate. Macerate with daily shaking for 1 to 2 weeks—constituents readily dissolve in this formula, which is designed to extract essential oils, mucilage, and tannins. The glycerine helps stabilize the tannins in solution, and augments the honeyed taste of the herb.

Water extracts: Basic tea of the dried, crushed flower cluster and bract. The herb is very light and fluffy. A heaping table-spoonful (1 g) may be steeped for 5 minutes in 1 cup of hot water. Strain and drink hot for the diaphoretic (sweat-inducing/fever reducing) effects. For cooling off on a hot day, sweeten the tea with honey and then pour over ice. The effect is refrigerant and diuretic.

Poultice: The fresh leaves of linden are loaded with healing mucilage and may be ground up or blended with a little water, applied in a thick layer to the affected area, and left on for half an hour or more. The linden leaf poultice treats wounds, sprains, and swellings. For easement of arthritic joints, briefly steam the leaves and apply hot, insulating with towels.

Practical uses: Sipping hot linden tea produces a marked vasodilating effect, bringing increased blood supply to the capillary bed. This causes an unusual degree of sweating, which in turn cools the body. Gentle enough for children and elders, and tasty enough to promote compliance, this is probably the best herbal treatment of all for helping bring down children's fevers. Administered with elderberry syrup, it can prove very useful in treatment of common cold and influenza. Given the loss of electrolytes through the sweat, once the patient has had a nap and starts to feel a bit better, they may be given a nice bowl of recuperation soup, well-salted.

The warm tea and tincture of linden flowers provides a relaxing nervine effect, and will serve to ease the mind and the musculature following a day of hard work and overstimulation. Take the tincture in a little water, drink the tea, or run your bath over a muslin bag containing 50 grams of dried linden flowers and steep yourself in it. The herb lowers the blood pressure and brings rapid, dreamless sleep. One awakens feeling positive and rested. Anyone with a propensity to uncontrolled spasm of leg muscles, which make even the most stolid warrior cry out "Uncle," are well-advised to take a little linden tea, which tends to banish the charley horse to the barn. The tea of linden bark, chopped and dried, helps detoxify the liver and is a good, gentle laxative.

Linden charcoal may be ground up and stirred into apple juice, being useful in treating runaway diarrhea and food poisoning. Effective dosage is 5 grams of linden carbon mixed into 1 cup of apple juice or similar carrier.

Dosage: According to basic recommendations found under "Dosage of tinctures," pages 49–52 and "Dosage of teas," pages 70–71. It is recommended that not more than the equivalent of the extractives of 2 grams of dried linden leaf be taken on a daily basis.

Contraindications: The prescribed dosage is generally safe for regular use by children and adults, even if pregnant or nursing. People suffering from heart problems or hypotension should not take this herb. The foliage of the tree may cause contact dermatitis among predisposed individuals. Breathing the pollen may result in an allergic response.

Other species: There are nearly 80 species in the Tilia genus, many of which are used in food, medicine, and woodworking. Our little-leaf lime (*Tilia cordata*) is among the finest, a stately tree native to Europe and commonly planted in cities worldwide—especially in France. The large-leaved lime (*Tillia platyphyllos*) is also commonly employed in medicine. Both species yield very tasty flowers and bracts.

Lobelia (Indian Tobacco) (*Lobelia inflata*)
Family: Bellflower (*Campanulaceae*)

Parts used: Entire plant, including stems, leaves, seedpods, and/or mature seed, best harvested in green seedpod stage. The herb may be used fresh or dried.

Acetous tincture of fresh herb: 1:5 (75A:25ACV)

Acetous tincture of dried herb or seed (preferred): 1:10 (50A:50ACV); see page 57–58.

Acetum: 1:7 (100ACV)

Practical uses: Among Americans, lobelia has gained a loyal following. It is not easy to administer correctly, due to the narrow window of correct dosage, yet the herb maintains its popularity. I believe this is simply because there is no better anti-spasmodic and expectorant available among the entire array of likely choices. Lobelia is of irreplaceable assistance in addressing chronic, debilitating cough and other lung-related problems, such as asthma and emphysema.

Dosage: This is a low-dose botanical. A dose of 5 drops of the acetous tincture taken 3 times daily (usually in marshmallow tea or with demulcent tinctures) should prove adequate. Lobelia tincture is generally combined with other tinctures at the rate of 1 part lobelia tincture by volume:9 parts of a mixture of other tinctures, such as: mullein, elecampane, thyme, hyssop, red root, or echinacea. This compound is taken at the basic dosage of 1 or 2 droppersful (30 to 60 drops), 3 to 5 times daily. Straight lobelia tinctures or compounds containing lobelia should be diluted in at least 1 full cup of water (240 ml) before ingestion. See "Compound cough syrup of spikenard," page 78.

Contraindications: Not to be taken during pregnancy. May cause nausea and vomiting. (Lobelia is an efficient emetic at high dosage.) Continuing to this day, there is a long-standing and unbroken tradition of Native Americans and later-day "Thomsonians" who intentionally take large doses of lobelia to purge the stomach. Overdose of the herb can temporarily affect the heart muscle, so those suffering from a weak heart or heart disease should avoid "lobelia puke" therapy.

Other species: Lobelia is a genus containing 350 species, many of them indigenous to America. Besides *Lobelia inflata*, several other species have been used historically for their medicinal attributes, including great blue lobelia (*L. siphilitica*), pale-spike lobelia (*L. spicata*), Kalm's lobelia (*L. kalmii*), and cardinal flower (*L. cardinalis*). These contain some of the same active alkaloids as *L. inflata*, which is nonetheless the preferred medicine.

Lomatium (*Lomatium dissectum*)
Family: Carrot (*Apiaceae)*

Parts used: The root of mature plants dug in the autumn and used fresh or dried. Wait until the fall rains soften the soil somewhat, and find the plants by way of their vestigial seed stalks. Take care when digging to preserve the root in whole form and undamaged. Roots bleed intensely aromatic, yellow-white oleo-gum-resin from every injury, and pieces left in the soil do not resprout. Briefly scrub the roots in cold water to remove soil and gravel, then dry them off before cutting up. For the purpose of fresh tincturing and making the infused oil, cut into 1-inch cubes. To prepare for dehydration, it is traditional to make horizontal slices through the root and dry these 1-inch thick, disc-like pieces whole. Dry on screens in a warm and airy place, turning frequently. Dried Lomatium slices are quite oily. They may be stored for up to a year in a sealed container at room temperature or cooler.

Tincture of fresh root: 1:2 (100A) Use Blender method, p.22. This makes a softly fibrous glop that is nonetheless easy to press.

Tincture of dried root: 1:5 (75A:25W) Crush the dried root pieces and soak overnight in the menstruum, then whip it up in a blender and macerate in the usual manner.

Oil, salve, or cream: Make infused herbal oil of the fresh root pieces. This can be used as-is or may be further processed into salve or cream (see "Chapter 10, Basic Formulas for Herbal Oils, Salves, and Creams," page 83, also pages 87–90).

Poultice of the fresh root: Cut up and smash the fresh root and apply to bruises, sprains, wounds, eruptions, or rheumatic joints.

Practical uses: The tincture, whether made from fresh or dried root, demonstrates strong antiviral and antibacterial activity. Lomatium has been used in treating viral hepatitis, mononucleosis, Epstein-Barr syndrome, HIV, asthma, pneumonia, colds, influenza, sore throat, tonsillitis, strep throat, staph infections, and amoebic dysentery. Both the oily products and the poultice soften the skin, dispel stuck blood, increase circulation to the affected area, fight infection, speed healing, and allay pain.

Dosage: This is a low dose botanical. Adult dosage is 5 to 10 drops mixed with 30 to 60 drops of dandelion tincture in half a glass of water, taken 3 times a day for a course of up to 10 days duration.

Contraindications: Highly sensitive individuals may experience the Lomatium rash side effect, consisting of reddish, raised, hive-like bumps that often occur on lower legs, thighs, at beltline, or on the back. If rash occurs, lower dosage or discontinue use. However, the condition may linger for several weeks before dissipating. Lomatium rash is annoying, but causes no lasting damage. Overdose of the tincture, or failure to combine with dandelion tincture as recommended, may result in a rash even in individuals not normally predisposed to allergies. Do not give Lomatium to children under the age of 10 (use black elderberry syrup instead).

Other species: *Lomatium* is a genus of up to 75 species of perennial herbs, of which our *L. dissectum* (fernleaf biscuitroot) is considered official. This plant may be differentiated from other species by the chocolate-brown umbel and the characteristically penetrating and antiseptic odor emanating from the swollen, smooth-skinned roots. *Lomatium macrocarpum, L. orientale, L utriculatum,* and especially *L. nudicaule* (barestem biscuitroot) have also been used by native healers in treating upper respiratory infection and gastrointestinal maladies.

Lovage (*Levisticum officinalis*)
Family: Carrot (*Apiaceae*)

Parts used: Entire plant consisting of the root, stems, and leaves, harvested prior to flowering and used fresh or dried. The seed harvested at maturity and dried.

Tincture of fresh herb: 1:2 (75A:25W)

Tincture of dried herb: 1:5 (50A:50W)

Tincture of seed: 1:4 (75A:25W)
The seeds can be ground up or bruised, soaked overnight in the menstruum, then briefly blended the following day and macerated in the usual manner.

Direct consumption: Chew the fresh leaves, the seed, or a small piece of the root.

Water extracts: Basic tea or decoction of any or all parts of the herb, fresh or dried.

Practical uses: Lovage is an aromatic stimulant to digestion and an antiflatulent. The weak tea is a good treatment for infant colic, administered by the teaspoonful. The tincture of the root or seeds is stronger than that made from other parts of the plant. This has been used as a substitute for dang-gui (*Angelica sinensis*), providing many of the same benefits. See "Dang-gui."

Dosage: According to basic recommendations found under "Dosage of tinctures," pages 49–52 and "Dosage of teas and decoctions," pages 70–71.

Poultice: The smooth leaves can be mashed or blended with a little water to make a cooling, healing poultice.

Food use: The fresh herb is a nutritive and carminative addition to soup, also imparting a celery-like flavor.

Contraindications: The strong tincture or decoction of root or seeds should not be taken during pregnancy. The stems and leaves are harmless. Prolonged usage or overdose of lovage can cause photosensitivity in predisposed individuals. Take care during harvest as exposure to the plant juices on sensitive skin areas followed by exposure to the sun may cause photosensitivity.

M

Ma-huang (*Ephedra sinica*)
Family: Joint Fir (*Ephedraceae*)

Part used: The jointed stem, harvested in the fall (when ephedrine content is at it highest) and dried. Store out of the light.

Tincture of dried herb: 1:5 (60A:30W:10ACV)
The above menstruum produces a balanced extract, taking into account the solvency of the main alkaloids present in ma-huang. Ephedrine is water- and alcohol-soluble, pseudoephedrine is alcohol-soluble, and *all* the ephedra alkaloids are better extracted by adding an acid (such as vinegar) to the menstruum (see pages 53–54). Store out of the light.

Water extract: Tea of the dried stem pieces (see "Dosage").

Practical uses: Ma-huang is one of the main Chinese herbs used to release the exterior, well-known to induce sweating, reduce wheezing, and promote urination. The herb is best used at the recommended dosage only as a palliative treatment for the common cold, influenza, asthma, and allergies. The herb dilates the bronchial passages while drying the mucous membranes of the upper respiratory tract—especially the sinuses.

Dosage: The basic tea is made with 3 grams of the herb taken in 3 doses over the course of 1 day. The tincture dosage is 10 to 30 drops taken 1 to 3 times per day.

Contraindications: Larger doses act as an adrenergic stimulant to the central nervous system, causing wakefulness and loss of hunger. Not to be taken for use during pregnancy or when nursing, by infants or the aged, or by those suffering from adrenal weakness, heart disease, thyroid imbalances, cardiac arrhythmia, high blood pressure, diabetes, thrombosis, or prostatitis. Not for use by those taking pharmaceutical MAOIs or heart medications. Overdose will result in lack of hunger, sleeplessness, elevated blood pressure, nervousness, tremors, psychosis, or even stroke.

Other species: Ma-huang (*Ephedra sinica*) is official, but two other species contain high levels of ephedrine alkaloids and are used interchangeably with the official drug. They are bluestem ephedra, mu-zei-ma-huang (*E. equisetina*), and zhong-ma-huang (*E. intermedia*). American *Ephedra* species are known as "Mormon tea." These include *E. californica, E. nevadensis,* and *E. viridis*, which act to dilate the bronchial passages without causing the stimulation associated with the Asian species.

Marshmallow (*Althaea officinalis*)
Family: Mallow (*Malvaceae*)

Parts used: Roots dug any time during the growth cycle or dormancy and used fresh or dried. Aerial parts of the plant, without the stems, harvested in early flower and used fresh or dried.

Tincture of fresh herb: 1:2 (50A:50W)

Tincture of dried herb: 1:5 (25A:75W)
Low or nonalcoholic extracts are preferred, because alcohol precipitates the healing mucilage, rendering highly-alcoholic extracts therapeutically useless.

Water extracts: The cold infusion of the fresh or dried leaf and/or flowers is the preferred preparation. Basic tea of the fresh or dried herb. Decoction of the dried root.

Direct consumption: A small piece of the sliced, dried root is slowly chewed. This is a specific remedy for ulcers.

Honeyed roots: Wash the young roots, then simmer in honey according to the directions on page 80. The honeyed roots are a delicious immune-enhancing and digestive tonic.

Practical uses: Marshmallow is a nutritive and immune-enhancing. This herb is one of the best agents employed for treating inflamed mucous membranes associated with colds, dry coughs, upper respiratory infection, urinary tract infection, and gastric or duodenal ulcer.

Dosage: According to basic recommendations found under "Dosage of tinctures," pages 49–52. In order to prevent precipitation of mucilage, do not combine marshmallow tincture with high-alcohol tinctures. The tea, decoction, or cold infusion may be taken freely without concern about overdose.

Poultice: The leaves may be lightly steamed and used as an application to swellings, infections, or chapped or dry skin. The roots can be mashed or cut in pieces and blended with a little water to make a cooling poultice for treating burns and new wounds. Alternately, the roots can be boiled until tender, mashed, and applied hot. This provides a more deep-seated influence and is a perfect anti-inflammatory treatment for swellings, puncture wounds, infected wounds, and splinters.

Contraindications: None known. Safe for general use. However, the coating action of the mucilage in marshmallow may delay absorption of other herbs or drugs.

Other species: Common mallow (*Malva neglecta*), high mallow *(M. sylvestris),* and even hollyhocks (*Alcea rosea*) have similar constituents to marshmallow and can be used interchangeably. However, the roots of these plants are generally woodier than marshmallow and are not very palatable as foods.

Meadowsweet
(*Spirea ulmaria* syn. *Filipendula ulmaria*)
Family: Rose (*Rosaceae*)

Parts used: The leaves and especially the flowers, without the stems, harvested in early flower and used fresh or dried.

Tincture of fresh herb: 1:2 (75A:15W:10Gly)

Tincture of dried herb: 1:5 (50A:40W:10Gly)

Water extracts: Basic tea of the fresh or dried herb.

Practical uses: The herb is generously endowed with salicylates, providing pain-relieving and anti-inflammatory activities against headache or muscular pain, colds, and flu. Taken very hot, the tea will help sweat out fevers, chills, and colds. Meadowsweet is also a valuable astringent, being particularly useful for treating infant diarrhea. Cool the tea before giving to infants. The honeyed aroma of the meadowsweet flower lifts the spirits and clears the head. The flowers can be used in brewing wine and beer.

Dosage: According to basic recommendations found under "Dosage of tinctures," pages 49–52 and "Dosage of teas and decoctions," pages 70–71.

Contraindications: None known. Safe for general use unless there is a specific allergy to salicylates. See "Willow."

Melilot (Sweet Clover) (*Melilotus officinalis*) Family: Legume (*Fabaceae*)

Parts used: Leaves and flowers, without the stems, harvested in early flower and used fresh, wilted, or dried.

Tincture of fresh or wilted herb: 1:2 (75A:25W)

Tincture of recently dried herb (preferred): 1:5 (50A:50W)

Water extract: Basic tea of dried herb.

Practical uses: Melilot is a blood thinner. The herb is a useful treatment for any condition of vascular congestion, including thrombophlebitis and hemorrhoids. Melilot also promotes digestion and, when taken after overeating, is a good antiflatulent.

Dosage: According to basic recommendations found under "Dosage of tinctures," pages 49–52 and "Dosage of teas and decoctions," pages 70-71.

External: As a wash or compress for treating varicose veins or ulcers, spider veins, or hemorrhoids, use the tea or dilute 2 droppersful of the tincture in 1 cup of cold water. Contraindications do not apply to the *external* use of melilot.

Poultice: The fresh leaves and flowers are bruised and laid on lymphatic swellings, painful varicosities, or on the breast as a treatment for mastitis.

Flavoring: Due to its pleasant aroma and digestive effects, the dried herb has been gainfully used for flavoring a variety of cheeses and liquors.

Contraindications: Not to be used during pregnancy. Melilot contains coumarin. Do not take with prescription drugs. This herb should not be taken in conjunction with the pharmaceutical anticoagulant warfarin, coumadin, or any preparations containing red clover (*Trifolium pratense*).

Other species: Melilot is a genus of 20 different species of plants. Our yellow-flowered sweet clover is used interchangeably with white-flowered sweet clover (*M. alba)*, which is so closely related that it is sometimes listed as a variety of the official species (i.e. *M. officinalis* var. *alba)*. The tall melilot (*M. altissima*) of Europe is also considered interchangeable with the official plant. Several other species are used as flavoring agents, food, and medicine in various parts of the world. These include *M. elegans* of the Mediterranean basin, *M. macrorhiza* of China and Asia, and *M. ruthenica* that hails from Russia.

Mint (Peppermint, Spearmint)
(*Mentha piperita, Mentha spicata*)
Family: Mint (*Lamiaceae*)

Part used: Entire fresh or dried aerial portions of the plant in flower, without the stems, used fresh or dried.

Tincture of fresh plant: 1:2 (100A)

Tincture of dried plant: 1:5 (75A:25W)

Glycerite of fresh plant: 1:2 (100Gly)

Water extract: Basic tea of the fresh or dried plant.

Practical uses: Mint is a universal flavoring agent that meets with enthusiastic acceptance by the general populace. The herb is used by itself, as a cooling, stimulating, and digestive beverage—soothing to the stomach. Mint can be combined with other herbs to improve their taste. The strong tea or tincture is the best cure ever for hiccups. The breath-freshening effects of mint make it the herb of choice for smokers.

Contraindications: The tea and tincture are safe for general use, but overindulgence can sometimes *cause* stomachache. Do not take if there is obstruction or inflammation of the bile ducts or the presence of bile stones. Avoid direct contact with pure, undiluted essential oil of mint, especially on sensitive skin, mucous membranes, and in eyes.

Other species: The genus *Mentha* is composed of at least 25 species that tend to naturally hybridize and intergrade. Besides peppermint and spearmint that are considered official, other distinct species demonstrating similar utility are water mint (*M. aquatica*), field mint (*M. arvensis*), and European horsemint (*M. longifolia*). European pennyroyal (*Mentha pulegium*) has similar effects, but is not recommended for use during pregnancy.

Motherwort (*Leonurus cardiaca*)
Family: Mint (*Lamiaceae*)

Parts used: Leaf and flowering tops, without the stems, harvested in very early flower and used fresh or dried. Seed harvested at maturity and dried.

Tincture of fresh herb: 1:2 (75A:25W)

Tincture of dried herb: 1:5 (50A:50W); see page 44.

Tincture of seed (very strong): 1:4 (75A:25W)
The seeds can be ground up or bruised, soaked overnight in the menstruum, then briefly blended the following day and macerated in the usual manner.

Water extracts: Basic tea of the fresh or dried herb. Decoction of the dried herb.

Syrup: Combine 1 part of the decoction of dried herb with 2 parts of honey by volume. The syrup has a calming influence and is used for the same purposes as the tincture, but is of marked advantage due to the improved taste. See "Chapter 9, Herbal Succi and Syrups," pages 77–78.

Practical uses: Motherwort brings on delayed menstruation and promotes regularity of the menstrual cycle. The herb strengthens and regulates heartbeat and regulates hyperactive thyroid.

Dosage: According to basic recommendations found under "Dosage of tinctures," pages 49–52 and "Dosage of teas and decoctions," pages 70–71.

Contraindications: Motherwort is clearly contraindicated for people exhibiting hypoactive thyroid.

Other species: Other species of this showy herb that are used in native medicine to regulate the blood include Siberian motherwort (*Leonurus sibericus*) and Chinese motherwort, (*L. artemisia*). The Pinyin name for this beauty is yi-mu-cao, literally "benefits mother herb."

Mullein (*Verbascum olympicum, V. thapsus*)
Family: Figwort (*Scrophulariaceae*)

Parts used: Fresh or dried leaf and/or flowers. The leaf is usually harvested in the first year, during the rosette stage. "Mullein flower" consists of the yellow flowers and sometimes includes the green calyx, but definitely does not include the entire woody stalk. The flowers are harvested at the peak of maturity, usually during the early summer of the second year of growth. Greek mullein (*V. olympicum*) presents flowers that can be readily stripped from the raceme, while flowers from common mullein (*V. thapsus*) must be picked individually—quite a chore.

Tincture of fresh leaf and/or flowers: 1:2 (50A:50W)

Tincture of dried leaf and/or flowers: 1:5 (25A:75W)
Mullein leaves take a long time to dry. They must be sliced across the midrib or slit up the midrib for faster drying. Leaves discolored by inefficient drying need to be composted. Mullein flowers are picked only after the morning dew has evaporated. Protect from bruising during the process of harvest and handling. Use an herb dryer with forced air set at 100° F (38° C). Once dried, the flowers can be tinctured immediately or mixed with other dried tea ingredients and stored in cellophane bags or glass jars.

Glycerite of fresh flowers: 1:2 (100Gly)

Water extracts: Tea of the fresh or dried flowers. Mullein flowers make a decorative and demulcent addition to tea blends, usually used in combination with other ingredients, such as marshmallow, *Echinacea purpurea* leaf and flower, elecampane root, etc.

Practical uses: Mullein is a soothing demulcent to the upper respiratory tract—gently astringent and expectorant. It is good for treating upper respiratory infection, cough, croup, sore throat, and bronchial catarrh. The combined demulcent and astringent effects make it a serviceable tea for treating mild diarrhea or infant diarrhea. There is a secondary nervine effect. The internal use of mullein will almost always prove mildly sedative.

Dosage: According to basic recommendations found under "Dosage of tinctures," pages 49–52 and "Dosage of teas and decoctions," pages 70–71. Also see "Dosage of glycerites, page 63."

Herbal oil: The infused oil of fresh mullein flowers is not only applicable for treating ear infection, but has a general emollient and antibacterial influence when used externally on any affliction of the skin, including: scrapes, cuts and infections, old burns, dry skin, and diaper rash. This oil can be used as an ingredient in healing salve (see "Basic Formulas for Herbal Salves," pages 87–90). Also see the formula and process for making ear oil under the "Garlic" heading in this formulary, page 178.

Poultice: Pick the large, fresh leaves from a mullein plant and steam actively until they are flexible, hot, and laden with water. Remove from the pot, cool slightly to tolerance, and lay directly on the affected area in several layers. Cover with a layer of plastic, insulate with towels or blankets, and leave to work for at least a half hour, or even overnight. This is good for shrinking ulcers, tumors, and glandular swellings, and is a specific treatment for mastitis—a treatment which, under other circumstances, would be quite fun.

Contraindications: None known. Safe for general use.

Smoking: The dried leaves can be smoked in a pipe or in rolling papers. The effect is to soothe the mucous membranes of the upper respiratory tract and lungs—an apparent contradiction of carrier and agent. Mullein used in this manner is probably safe for occasional use. Mullein leaves are sometimes added to traditional smoking mixtures, which may also contain leaves or floweres of coltsfoot, motherwort, Scotch broom, tobacco, uva-ursi, willow, wilde dagga, and the like.

N

Nettles (Stinging Nettles) (*Urtica dioica*)
Family: Nettle (*Urticaceae*)

Parts used: Entire aerial parts (stem and leaf) of young plants, harvested in the spring and used fresh or dried. Fresh dormant roots. Seed harvested in early maturity, along with the persistent green calyx, and dried.

Tincture of fresh plant or root: 1:2 (75A:25W)

Tincture of dried plant or seed: 1:5 (50A:50W)

Water extracts: Basic tea of the fresh or dried herb. Cold infusion of the fresh or dried herb. Decoction of the dried herb or seeds.

Succus: In the spring, harvest the entire fresh nettle plant, mash or blend it, then express the juice with a tincture press. Combine 1 part alcohol by volume:3 parts nettle juice by volume (see "Chapter 9, Herbal Succi and Syrups").

Practical uses: Legion. The herb is a nutritive spring tonic, blood builder, and blood cleanser, high in chlorophyll, calcium, and potassium. Use of nettles bolsters the entire body and improves resistance to allergens, including environmental pollutants, molds, and pollen. The tincture of the fresh roots is a specific anti-inflammatory for treating prostatitis. The fresh herb can be used in making beer, delivering the salutary effects in a most agreeable vehicle.

Dosage: According to basic recommendations found under "Dosage of tinctures," pages 49–52 and "Dosage of teas and decoctions," pages 70–71.

Hair tonic: The decoction of the dried herb, and especially the seeds, stimulates hair growth, helps restore balding hair, and improves the overall texture and tone of the hair. Use the decoction as a wash after shampooing and leave on for at least 3 minutes before rinsing off.

Flagellation: For treating arthritic joints, whipping with fresh, mature nettles will stimulate circulation to the swollen area, relieve pain, and greatly increase freedom of movement. Although some people cannot tolerate this heroic therapy, others find that the initial shock gives way to a pleasant buzzing sensation followed by 2 or more days of freedom from pain and inflammation. This therapy should be approached with circumspection.

Food use: Fresh spring nettles are lightly steamed to disarm the stinging hairs and eaten as a tonic. They are like spinach. The water remaining after simmering or steaming nettles is a special treat for the cook, taken warm by the cupful while working in the kitchen.

Contraindications: Fresh nettles are armed with stinging hairs, actually phytohypodermic needles that inject irritating formic acid into the skin on contact. Depending on the individual constitution, this may be perceived either as a "sting" or as "stimulation." The antidote to this stinging is usually growing close by—yellow dock leaf, jewelweed, mint, rosemary, or sage. Worry the leaf until it becomes juicy, then rub into the affected area. A paste made of baking soda and water will also relieve the stinging. Overindulgence in nettle tea or decoction can result in a condition called "urticaria," where transient, painfully itchy, red wheals erupt on the skin. If this occurs, discontinue use of the nettles, drink plenty of water, and the condition will eventually disappear. Violet tea or tincture, or slippery elm bark, taken internally and used externally, will help speed the resolution of urticaria. Avoid internal use of nettle products made of mature (summer or fall) leaf, due to the presence of tiny cystoliths (calcium carbonate concretions) that may irritate the kidneys and encourage formation of urinary stone. Using the tincture of nettle root sometimes produces mild gastrointestinal upset.

Other species: There are 80 species in the Urtica genus, ranging worldwide and widely used in manufacture of fiber and in medicine. Roman nettles (*Urtica pilulifera*) are native to southern Europe, but were transported north by Roman soldiers, who purportedly flagellated themselves to keep warm. Annual nettle (*U. urens*) is used interchangeably with our *U. dioica.* The seeds of annual nettle are particularly large and tasty.

O

Oats (*Avena sativa*)
Family: Grass (*Poaceae*)

Part used: For herbal use, the green seed is harvested in the immature "milky" stage and used fresh or dried. The test for readiness is to take one of the swollen fruits (seeds) and compress it between the thumbnails. If a milky sap exudes, then the seed is ready to be harvested, either for fresh tincturing or to dry for later use. The seeds are simply stripped from the stalk by hand. For food use, the grain is harvested when mature and dry.

Tincture of fresh, milky seed: 1:2 (75A:25W)

Water extracts: Basic tea or decoction of the fresh or dried, immature seed.

Practical uses: Oat seed is a gentle nervine tonic for treating exhaustion, sleeplessness, adrenal burnout, or addiction to nicotine, caffeine, or other drugs. The herb is also a serviceable diuretic.

Food use: Oatmeal, when eaten as a cooked bowl of porridge or as a raw cereal (Swiss-style muesli) provides significant health advantages beyond good taste and nutrition. Oatmeal is full of soluble fiber (beta-glucan) which helps reduce the level of low-density lipoproteins (LDL), or "bad" cholesterol in the human body. This translates to a lower risk of atherosclerosis, which in turn reduces the likelihood of high blood pressure and cardiovascular disease, heart attack, and stroke. The operable dosage appears to be a bowl of oatmeal taken at least 6 times per week.

Dosage: According to basic recommendations found under "Dosage of tinctures," pages 49–52 and "Dosage of teas and decoctions," pages 70–71.

Contraindications: None known. Safe for general use.

Other species: Cultivated oats (*Avena sativa*) has been selected over the past two millennia from various wild oats including *A. barbata, A. fatua,* and *A. sterilis.* The wild species are medicinally interchangeable with the cultivated form.

Oregano (*Origanum* spp.)
Family: Mint (*Lamiaceae*)

Parts used: Leaves and/or flowers and bracts without the stems, harvested in flowering stage and used fresh or dried.

Tincture of fresh herb: 1:2 (100A)

Tincture of dried herb: 1:5 (75A:25W)

Acetum of dried herb: 1:7 (100ACV)

Water extract: Basic tea of the fresh or dried herb.

Practical uses: Used medicinally, oregano has broad activity as an antioxidant (cell-protector), antiseptic, preservative, anthelmintic, and antifungal. The tea or tincture can be taken for treating virally or bacterially mediated colds and upper respiratory infections. The essential oils exert an antiseptic influence on the lungs, bronchi, and nasal passages.

Dosage: According to basic recommendations found under "Dosage of tinctures," pages 49–52, "Dosage of dry herb aceta," pages 55–56, and "Dosage of teas and decoctions," pages 70–71.

Food use: The herb is a classic spice for pizza, and the anti-oxidant effects are important in the presence of oils and fats baked at high temperatures.

Contraindications: None known. Safe for general use. Avoid direct contact with pure, undiluted essential oil of oregano, especially on sensitive skin, mucous membranes, and in eyes.

Other species: Greek oregano (*O. heracleoticum*) and its several cultivars (e.g. Italian oregano and Sicilian oregano) are useful medicinally and are also excellent for food use. Sweet marjoram (*O. majorana*) is fruity, being used almost exclusively as a culinary spice. The herb zaatar (*O. syriacum*) is fluffy and tasty, an ingredient in the traditional Middle Eastern condiment of the same name.

Recipe for zaatar: Combine ¼ cup zaatar leaf, 2 tablespoons ground sumac berries, ¼ cup toasted sesame seeds, and 1 tablespoon coarse sea salt. Rub together until thoroughly mixed. Sometimes garlic is added. Eat with olive oil and bread.

234

Oregon Grape (*Mahonia* spp.)
Family: Barberry (*Berberidaceae*)

Parts used: The root, or preferably the root bark, dug in the autumn or winter and used fresh or dried. Dig the roots and wash them, then cut into ½ inch pieces with snips. To make the root bark, take whole, washed roots and whittle thin quills of the root bark from the inner wood. Combining the root with a small amount of leaf prior to extraction will produce a more effective tincture. This is due to the efflux pump inhibitors found in the aerial parts of the plant, which synergize with the root alkaloids to disarm gram-positive bacteria. Use 4 parts root to 1 part leaves and tincture as per below:

Tincture of fresh root (with leaves if possible): 1:2 (60A:40W)

Tincture of dried root (with leaves if possible): 1:5 (50A:50W)

Water extract: Basic tea of the fresh or dried root bark. Decoction of the dried root.

Practical uses: Oregon grape is a valuable digestive tonic, incorporating the triple functions of bitter tonic, mild liver stimulant, and antibacterial agent in one herb. The main indications for its use are indigestion (especially poor fat or protein metabolism), oily or dry skin with acne or psoriasis, coated tongue with bad breath, chronic constipation, and bacterial infection. The herb stimulates secretions, tonifies the mucous membranes, helps build blood, and moves the lymph. Oregon grape serves as a prophylactic and curative for traveler's diarrhea caused by the exotic bacteria that accompany unfamiliar food and water.

Dosage: According to basic recommendations found under "Dosage of tinctures," pages 49–52 and "Dosage of teas and decoctions," pages 70–71. Given the digestive bitter aspects of the herb, it makes sense to take the tea or tincture just prior to meals.

Contraindications: Do not use when *chronic* gastrointestinal irritation or inflammation (such as excessive salivation, red tongue, and irritable bowel) predominate—it is counterproductive to stimulate metabolic processes that are already in an excited state.

Other species: Tall Oregon grape (*Mahonia aquifolium*) is not only the official species, but also the easiest to grow, given its preference for full sun and garden soils. However, all types of Oregon grape, including the creeping forms (*M. nervosa*, *M. repens)*, and California barberry (*M. pinnata*) are interchangeable in medicine.

Osha (Bear Medicine) (*Ligusticum porteri*) Family: Carrot (*Apiaceae*)

Parts used: The root is the part most commonly employed in herbal medicine, smokey-smelling, dark-skinned, and convoluted, showing characteristic yearly growth rings below the crown, rimmed with upturned, hair-like fibers that are vestige of the leaf stems of previous years. The roots are dug in the fall, briefly scrubbed in water, then used fresh or sun-dried. Drying in the sun does not diminish their medicinal activity. Whole, dried roots or root pieces may be stored in a sealed container. Osha roots retain their potency for years.

Tincture of dry root: 1:5 (70A:30W) The active constituents in osha are only partially water-soluble. Therefore, the alcoholic tincture of the dried root is really the preferred preparation.

Direct consumption: A small piece of the fresh or dried root is held in the mouth and slowly chewed. This is a good practice for treating sore throat, as the antiseptic and anesthetic resins are slowly and soothingly released.

Honeyed roots: Fresh osha roots are scrubbed, sliced thinly, and simmered in honey, which substantially improves their taste without much compromising their medicinal activity (see page 80).

Osha syrup: Fresh osha roots are scrubbed, sliced thinly, and packed in a quart jar, then covered with honey and allowed to sit in the sun. Cover the jar with cheesecloth, held tightly over the top by screwing on the canning ring. This allows the liquid to evaporate out of the roots without condensing on the lid, which helps keep the syrup from going bad. After a week, the essence of osha will have been taken up by the honey. Uncap and pour the lot through several layers of cheesecloth, collecting the medicated honey in another jar. Store in the refrigerator and use by the tablespoonful, as needed, for treating the common cold, flu, bronchitis, or sore throat.

Practical uses: Osha is a powerful vasodilator. A dropperful of the tincture taken in hot tea will help produce a good sweat, which brings down the fever of colds and flu. Osha fights bacteria and viruses that cause upper respiratory infection, and helps eliminate toxins. The herb is a reasonable antitussive, and combines well with soothing herbs such as licorice, marshmallow, and slippery elm, all of which serve to make coughs more productive and therefore less long-lived. Osha is also a powerful bronchodilator, widening the large-bore air passages leading from the trachea to the lungs, stimulating the ciliated cells to bring up and expunge metabolic debris. Increased air supply to the lungs is generally helpful on a hike, and especially a hike at altitude. The improved air intake and slower heart rate will help dispel the headache, dizziness, and nausea associated with altitude sickness. Lacking coca, chew osha!

Dosage: Osha tincture is very strong. Take 10-30 drops 3 times a day, or use 3-drop doses, well-diluted in water, as needed for treating cough. Children do best with the candied roots or syrup.

Contraindications: Not to be used during pregnancy.

Other species: There are three species of *Ligusticum* that are used interchangeably in local herbal medicine. They can be successfully promoted by intentionally reseeding the wilds and by growing them in the domestic garden. These include our osha (*L. porteri*) of the Rocky Mountains, fernleaf licorice-root (*L. filicinum*) which is a more northerly ranging species, and Gray's licorice-root (*L. grayi*) which inhabits a more westerly range and is quite familiar to me here in the Siskiyou Mountains of Southern Oregon. None of these useful plants should ever be confused with poison hemlock (*Conium maculatum*). Let the wild digger beware! The roots of poison hemlock are inodorous and lack the characteristic crown of fibers that distinguishes true osha from toxic look-alikes. Cultivate and dig the osha, but leave the conium—alone-ium.

Passionflower (*Passiflora incarnata*)
Family: Passionflower (*Passifloraceae*)

Parts used: Succulent vines, leaves, and flower buds harvested in early flower and used fresh or dried. The constituents of this quirky plant will differ according to the season of harvest, and the active flavonoids seem to be at their highest concentration and best stability during the early flowering stage.

Tincture of fresh herb: 1:2 (75A:25W)

Tincture of dry herb: 1:5 (50A:50W)

Water extracts: Basic tea or decoction.

Practical uses: Passionflower slows the pulse and sedates. The herb can lessen nerve pain, painful menses, and headache, and is most effective for treating nervous restlessness and insomnia. For light sleepers, and if there is a tendency toward bad dreams, passionflower will deepen the sleep and usually brings good dreams. The herb combines well with valerian, augmenting the sedative effects and banishing "valerian nightmares." However, I feel compelled to temper these statements with that of Shaban, a very handsome and jet black half-Somali who cooked for us when we lived in East Africa. He was standing in the kitchen one day when I bit into an aromatic yellow passion fruit. Shaban said *"Italeta utaota mbaya sana,"* which loosely translated from the Swahili means, "That will bring you very bad dreams." On further investigation, however, I learned that Shaban considered all dreaming to be bad dreaming. Passionflower, in all its guises, begs to be considered in cultural context . . .

Dosage: According to basic recommendations found under "Dosage of tinctures," pages 49–52 and "Dosage of teas and decoctions," pages 70–71.

Contraindications: None known. Safe for general use.

Other species: *Passiflora* is a genus containing about 400 species demonstrating various degrees of potency and sometimes doubtful edibility and biological activities. Furthermore, passionflower tends to hybridize naturally in the wild, and the chemistry of a given species will vary from region to region. Not all *Passiflora* species are medicinally interchangeable or useful, and therefore it makes sense to utilize the "official" variety (i.e. *P. incarnata*), which has been well-tested and is generally dependable. The leaf of purple passionflower (*P. edulis*), a species that bears larger, tastier fruits than *P. incarnata*, is also fairly commonly used for making the sedative medicine.

Pepper, Cayenne
(*Capsicum frutescens* syn. *C. annuum*)
Family: Nightshade (*Solanaceae*)

Part used: Whole red peppers, with or without the seeds, used fresh or dried.

Tincture of fresh peppers: 1:2 (100A)

Tincture of dried peppers: 1:5 (75A:25W)

Capsules: Depending on sensitivity, as little as ½ "00" capsule or as many as 2 "00" capsules of the dried ground peppers may be taken with a cup of water. The advantage of the capsule, in this case, is for people who cannot tolerate the pungency of cayenne, but are in practical need of it. The capsule carries the herb deeper into the intestines, where it best does its antidiarrheal work.

Practical uses: Cayenne is used for strengthening the heart muscle and for increasing circulation. In emergency situations—such as heart failure—cayenne tincture can be administered to stimulate the heart muscle, restore active circulation, and normalize blood pressure. Used during or after meals, cayenne promotes gastric secretions and assists in digestion. The herb is commonly employed for treating cold extremities and the common cold. In the case of diarrhea caused by exotic bacteria, cayenne will often promote a rapid return to normal gastrointestinal function. The herb may be taken as a part of a daily diet, to ward off disease in general and specifically to act as a prophylactic against cancer.

Dosage: Of the capsule, up to 3 times per day, during or after meals. Of the tincture, 10 to 20 drops in a full glass of water, taken 3 times per day, during or after meals.

External: As a rubefacient, the tincture may be diluted with 2 parts of grain alcohol or rubbing alcohol and massaged into the skin. This brings a warm glow to tired muscles or rheumatic joints, improving circulation and relieving pain. Try this on a small area to start with, in order to judge tolerance levels. The sensation of heat may build for some minutes.

Food use (recipe for hot sauce):
>   You will need:
>   ½ lb of fresh cayenne peppers
>   6 cloves of fresh garlic
>   1 teaspoon salt
>   1 cup apple cider vinegar

One of the easiest and tastiest of hot sauces relies on roasted peppers. Heat a cast iron skillet on medium heat until hot, then spread the fresh peppers in the pan, enough to cover the bottom surface, but not so many that they stack up. Turn the peppers occasionally, until they are fragrant, wilted, and develop blackened spots. If the peppers start to smoke profusely or char, turn down the heat. A well-roasted pepper should be soft and juicy. If you have a lot of peppers and a big appetite for sauce, increase the above recipe, and roast the peppers in batches. Put the hot peppers in a paper bag and allow them to cool before proceeding. Leave the husks on the garlic cloves and roast in much the same manner, until the insides are soft. Once the garlic has cooled, it is easy to remove the husks. Place the garlic, peppers, and salt in a non-reactive pan or bowl, add the vinegar, and leave covered overnight. The next morning, boil the mixture briefly (5 minutes). Cool the mixture and blend to a smooth puree in a blender. Given the preservative effect of capsaicin, garlic, and vinegar, the bottled sauce will store in the refrigerator for 3 months or more. Cayenne is a culinary herb of high repute, making even the blandest of foods taste pungent and savory.

Contraindications as below:

External: Although contact with cayenne herb or extract will not permanently damage the eyes or mucous membranes, it can cause serious discomfort. If cayenne gets into the eyes or mucous membranes, flush freely with cold water or milk until the burning abates. If skin contact with cayenne causes uncomfortable burning, rinse first with plain rubbing or grain alcohol and then wash with soap and water.

Internal: Excessive dosage may cause gastrointestinal discomfort in sensitive individuals. Cayenne should not be used if there is inflammation of the mucous membranes or excessive discharge of mucous, as the herb will tend to exacerbate this condition.

Processing cautions: Cayenne should be handled with great respect and kept out of the eyes and mucous membranes. Always wear a filter mask when grinding dried cayenne. Machinery used to process cayenne must be cleaned with alcohol, then soap and water, or the potent oils and resins will be detectable in subsequent products. Manufacturing herbalists usually keep a tincture press hose aside, dedicated to cayenne use only. This helps prohibit transfer of pungent oils from one product to another.

Other species: The taxonomy of the *Capsicum* genus is complicated and confused, probably as a result of the long history of selection which has differentiated many varieties of peppers (e.g. African bird, chili, sweet bell, habanero, pimento, paprika, tabasco, Thai, etc.). *Capsicum baccatum*, a relatively obscure group of peppers native to Bolivia and Peru, are fast-growing and tolerant of cold conditions. *Criolla sella* is probably the most well-known of these, making flat-topped bushes studded copiously with 3-inch, golden-orange, moderately hot peppers that may be harvested even after the first frost. Cayenne itself is readily recognized by its characteristically thin, long pods and extreme pungency, owing to the high concentration of a compound known as capsaicin. Perhaps this is why cayenne, which performs consistently and dependably in cultivation, is regarded as official. As long as they taste pungent, other varieties of peppers may be substituted for cayenne "in a pinch."

241

Plantain (*Plantago lanceolata, P. major*)
Family: Plantain (*Plantaginaceae*)

Parts used: Leaf and stem harvested spring through fall and used fresh or dried. Seed harvested at maturity and dried.

Tincture of fresh herb (preferred): 1:2 (75A:25W)

Tincture of dried herb: 1:5 (50A:50W)

Water extracts: Basic tea of the fresh or dried herb. Basic decoction of the dried herb. Cold infusion, tea, or decoction of the seeds.

Succus: Harvest the entire fresh plantain plant in the spring, mash or blend, then express the juice in a tincture press. Preserve by adding 1 part alcohol by volume: 3 parts plantain juice by volume. See "Chapter 9, Herbal Succi and Syrups," pages 73–75.

Practical uses: Plantain is a spring tonic, a gentle alterative, antiseptic, and astringent. The uses are legion, including the treatment of toothache, infections, cough, diarrhea, and hemorrhoids. Plantain is a specific for treating skin problems, such as eczema or acne. The seeds contain huge amounts of mucilage and are a direct and oft-employed substitute for psyllium, demonstrating the same emollient and laxative effects. These should always be taken with ample quantities of water.

Dosage: According to basic recommendations found under "Dosage of tinctures," pages 49–52 and "Dosage of teas and decoctions," pages 70–71.

External: To treat skin problems, plantain may be taken internally and also used externally as a wash or compress. Use the tea, succus, plant juice, or full strength tincture.

Poultice: The bruised or mashed leaves make an excellent drawing poultice. Applied as a thick mash, this is a useful application to splinters, infections, eczema, oily skin, acne, and especially toothache and abscess. To make a pulling poultice for dental application, mash the leaves and wrap in 1 or 2 layers of clean cheesecloth or gauze, shaping a small bolus. This can be placed between the inner lip and the offending tooth or swollen gum.

Food use: As a boy scout I read that plantain is one of the best of all survival foods. Hiking the rolling green hills and hardwood forests along the Iowa River with my "Boy Scout Handbook" in hand, I picked the largest, most mature leaves of broadleaf plantain I could find. These I washed in a little water from my canteen, then boiled in the classic aluminum pot suspended over a smoky fire of oak twigs. But even after trying "several changes of water" to dispel the astringency, the leaves were not quite edible. I determined then that consumption of plantain as a vegetable should be relegated strictly to starvation situations. Later, I discovered that the *very young* leaves were palatable. My handbook must have been written by an armchair survivalist and did not mention to pick the young leaves instead of the old. The two species of sea plantain (*Plantago maritima and P. decipiens*), which are salty and stringless, are the tastiest of them all.

Contraindications: None known. Safe for general use.

Other species: The English plantain (*Plantago lanceolata*) and the broad-leaved plantain (*P. major*) are considered official, but there are several other species that can be used interchangeably with them. This includes goosetongue, the halophytic sea plantain *(P. maritima)*, which is native to maritime Europe, Russia, Greenland, and the Atlantic and Pacific coasts of North America. Herba stella (*P. coronopus*) of Eurasia, Chinese plantain (*P. asiatica*), and ispaghul (*P. amplexicaulis*) of tropical Asia and Arabia have been used to produce the "psyllium seed" of commerce. The psyllium plant (*P. psyllium*), which is native to the Mediterranean basin, has hairy leaves that are not much used in medicine. However, this plant produces the highest quality seed—rich in mucilage and fatty acids.

Adulteration: In Europe, wild-harvested plantain has been known to contain the leaf of Greek foxglove (*Digitalis lanata*) as an adulterant. In the early stages of growth, these two plants really do look very much alike. This is clearly a dangerous situation, when an herb containing cardiac glycosides is mixed with a harmless herb like plantain. Domestic cultivation of the herb reduces the possibility of misidentification.

Pleurisy Root (Butterfly Weed) (*Asclepias tuberosa*)
Family: Milkweed (*Asclepiadaceae*)

Part used: Root of 2-year-old or older plants harvested during dormancy and dried.

Tincture of the dried root: 1:5 (50A:50W)

Water extracts: Basic tea or decoction of the ground or finely sliced, dried root.

Practical uses: Pleurisy root promotes sweating and the expulsion of toxic metabolic waste through the sweat. The herb reduces inflammation of dry mucous membranes and serous membranes, generally used to treat acute and severe symptoms of fever, pneumonia, pleurisy, bronchitis, asthma, cough, or diarrhea.

Dosage: Of the tincture, 5 to 15 drops taken up to 3 times a day. Of the tea and decoction, half the standard dosage as found under "Dosage of teas and decoctions," pages 70–71.

Contraindications: Not to be used during pregnancy. The use of fresh (undried) pleurisy root, or overdose of the dried root, is likely to cause nausea and vomiting. Not for extended use.

Poke (*Phytolacca americana* syn. *P. decandra*)
Family: Poke (*Phytolaccaceae*)

Parts used: Root dug during dormancy. New spring leaves or ripe berries. The dried root is considered inferior to the fresh root or berries.

Tincture of fresh root or berries: 1:2 (75A:25W).

Practical uses: Poke is a lymphatic stimulant used for resolving glandular blockage and helping dispel metabolic waste products. It is not a substance to use lightly and is best employed to treat people who are very ill—especially when gentler therapies fail.

Dosage: Poke is a low-dose botanical. Maximum adult dosage of the fresh root or berry tincture is 6 drops well-diluted in at least 1 full cup of water (240 ml), taken up to 3 times daily. See "Contraindications."

Infused oil of fresh poke root (TOXIC):

1) Dig the root, scrub it well, and dry it off.
2) Cut in thin (¼ inch = .64 cm), diagonal slices and pack these into a wide-mouth glass pint or quart canning jar.
3) Cover the root slices with organic olive oil, and place the jar in a very warm location (~110° F = ~43° C), such as an herb dryer on "high" or in an oven set at 100° F. It is advisable to keep the jar in a bread pan or other shallow tray containing a small amount of warm, insulating water on the off possibility that the jar might break in the night and cause a huge mess or even start a fire.
4) After 2 days, remove the jar from this gentle heat and affix cheesecloth over the mouth, securing it with a rubber band. Then pour the oil through the cheesecloth into another jar, leaving the fresh root slices behind. These can be composted.
5) Allow the crude oil to sit undisturbed overnight, then decant through cheesecloth again, taking care to exclude any water droplets that may be lurking on the bottom of the settling jar.
6) The finished oil is bottled in amber glass and marked prominently with the universally understood symbol of skull and crossbones and the words: **Toxic. Poke Oil. For external use only.**
7) Store out of the light in a cool place.

The oil will last for at least a year. Poke oil is a specific remedy for application to glandular swellings, including swollen lymph in the neck, underarm or groin, and the breast, in the case of mastitis. If treating a nursing mother, the oil is applied after nursing and thoroughly washed from the nipple area prior to the next nursing. This therapy can be supported by intermittently applying a poultice of hot mullein leaf or steamed, mashed marshmallow root or leaf (see Chapter 11, "Poultices, Compresses, and Soaks").

Food use: The tender, young leaves or "spreens" (spring greens) of poke are a traditional food in the southern and midwestern states of North America. They are very good, but must not be eaten fresh (uncooked). The leaves are usually simmered in 2 changes of water, in order to leach out toxic substances prior to consumption, but some people eat them fried or pickled without leaching. Regardless of the degree of pretreatment, there is little doubt that poke spreens lend an alterative, laxative, blood-cleansing, and lymphatic influence.

Contraindications as below:

Internal: No parts of the plant (including the appetizing-looking berries!) should be ingested without proper preparation and dosage. Warn children not to eat the berries. Not for use during pregnancy. Use only under the guidance of a qualified health professional. Some people are sensitive to poke and will develop a rash. If this occurs, reduce dosage or discontinue use. Overdose of poke will cause loose stools and general gastrointestinal upset, and may cause drastic purging.

External application of poke oil is usually well-tolerated. If a slight redness or rash occurs, this is a sign of stimulation and is no cause for alarm. If a pimply rash develops, discontinue use or dilute the poke oil with equal parts of olive oil, and/or use only once daily until the problem is resolved.

Other species: There are 25 species in the *Phytolacca* genus, several of which are used similarly to American poke as foods and as alterative medicines. These include Tibetan poke (*Phytolacca acinosa*), gopo berry (*P. abyssinica*) of East Africa, bella sombra (*P. dioica*) of Argentina, and Venezuela pokeberry (*P. rivinoides*) of tropical America.

Poppy, California
(*Eschscholzia californica*)
Family: Poppy (*Papaveraceae*)

Parts used: Root, leaf, flowers, and seedpods harvested in late flowering/early seeding stage and used fresh or dried.

Tincture of fresh plant: 1:2 (75A:25W)

Tincture of dried plant: 1:5 (50A:50W)

Water extract: Basic tea of dried plant.

Practical uses: California poppy is a sedative, especially useful for treating anxiety and restlessness. The herb serves as a pain reliever for body, head, and toothaches and, in many cases, will induce a deep and dreamless sleep. It is mild enough for treating children, sensitive individuals, and the aged.

Dosage: Basic adult dosage is 1 cup of the tea or 30 drops of the tincture, taken once or twice before bedtime. The dosage is halved for treating children.

Contraindications: Not to be used during pregnancy or in conjunction with pharmaceutical monoamine oxidase inhibitors (MAOIs). Not recommended for treating infants. Overdose can cause headache and general body malaise the day following use.

Other species: There are at least eight different species in the *Eschscholzia* genus native to the American Southwest. These hybridize in nature and are therefore often difficult to differentiate. They are characterized by a long, tapering seedpod with a basal ring. Although it is likely that they all contain protopine alkaloids, the efficacy and safety of these various species, and the numerous horticultural varieties that have been developed from them, has not been well-established. Therefore, it makes sense to grow and utilize the typical orange and yellow flowered, wild California poppy (*Eschscholzia californica*).

Pulsatilla (*Anemone pulsatilla*)
Family: Crowfoot (*Ranunculaceae*)

Parts used: Whole plant harvested in flowering stage, either including or excluding the root, and used fresh. The dried herb is nearly inert.

Tincture of fresh plant: 1:2 (75A:25W)

Practical uses: Pulsatilla is a powerful nervine and antispasmodic, generally used for treating women, especially those with light or wan complexions, poor circulation, high blood pressure, and low nerve force. The indications are nervous exhaustion, shock, headache, and nerve pain, or PMS symptoms with worry and depression. The action of the herb is to slow and strengthen the pulse, improve circulation, banish depression, and bring healing sleep.

Dosage: This is a low-dose botanical. The starting adult dosage is 5 to 10 drops diluted in a full glass of water, taken twice daily.

Contraindications: Not to be used during pregnancy or for those with low blood pressure. For adults only. The herb should be used only under the care and direction of a qualified health professional. Symptoms of overdose are gastric distress, nausea, low blood pressure, eruptive rash, and in rare cases convulsions.

Processing cautions: Cutting and grinding or blending of fresh pulsatilla should be carried out in a well-ventilated area. The fresh herb, seeds, and the tincture of the fresh herb can be irritating or downright caustic to the skin, mucous membranes, and eyes. I once contracted a huge, painful, fluid-filled blister on the thigh by keeping pulsatilla seeds in my pocket during a hike.

Other species: Pulsatilla is known by the common names pasqueflower or windflower, represented by about 33 species worldwide. *Anemone canadensis, A hirsutissima, A. occidentalis, A. patens, A. pratensis,* etc. all have some degree of activity. However, given that members of this genus are potentially quite toxic, it makes sense to grow and use the purple-flowered *Anemone pulsatilla*, which is official.

Purslane (*Portulaca oleracea*)
Family: Purslane (*Portulacaceae*)

Parts used: Leaves and stems harvested in vegetative or early flowering stage and used fresh.

Tincture of fresh herb: 1:2 (50A:50W)

Succus: Grind or mash the fresh herb and express the juice in a tincture press. Use 1 part alcohol by volume:3 parts expressed juice. See "Chapter 9, Herbal Succi and Syrups," pages 73–75.

Acetum: Keep leaves and stems whole, or chop coarsely and pack them in a jar, sprinkle liberally with salt, and cover with apple cider vinegar. These are eaten later as pickles.

Direct consumption: In season, the best way to take the herb is directly from the garden or field, chewed slowly and savored.

Practical uses: Purslane is a nutritive, vitamin-rich, digestive and urinary tonic, full of mucilage and containing more Omega-3 fatty acids than any other terrestrial plant. The herb is also used to treat fevers and sunstroke. As a demulcent to the urinary tract, purslane is good for treating scanty or burning urine.

Dosage: According to basic recommendations found under "Dosage of tinctures," pages 49–52.

Poultice: The fresh, mashed leaves make a cooling and healing poultice for soothing inflammation of the eyes or skin, old ulcerations, burns, or infected cuts.

Food use: The fresh leaves are best used in salads with other ingredients. They can also be boiled or steamed and eaten as a vegetable, or added to stir-fry and soup.

Contraindications: None known. Safe for general use.

Other species: The *Portulaca* genus is represented by nearly 100 different species growing worldwide, generally consisting of thick-leaved and mucilaginous bedding plants. There are several other species used as food and medicine, including chicken-weed purslane (*P. quadrufida*) of Africa and yellow purslane (*P. lutea*) of Polynesia. Golden purslane (*P. oleracea* var. *sativa*) is the tasty, cultivated form.

Red Root (*Ceanothus americanus, C. velutinas*)
Family: Buckthorn (*Rhamnaceae*)

Parts used: Woody root, including the root bark, used fresh or dried. The leaves and twigs, used fresh or dried.

Tincture of fresh root: 1:2 (65A:25W:10Gly)
Roots exhibiting the most red coloration are the best for making medicine. Snip or whittle the root immediately after digging and washing. The dryer it gets, the more it becomes like herbal steel. Will it grind in a blender? Don't even think of it.

Tincture of dried root: 1:5 (50A:40W:10Gly)
The root and root bark are reduced to very small pieces when fresh, then dried on screens and ground in a hammer mill to a coarse powder. Large pieces of the roots will eat the hammer mill alive. Macerate for 5 weeks in order to accomplish full extraction.

Water extracts: Tea of the dried leaves. Decoction of the dried root pieces.

Practical uses: The root tincture of red root is a stimulant to the lymph (somewhat of a nontoxic substitute for poke), an effective and time-honored remedy for relieving mild congestion of the glandular system, liver, and spleen. The herb also shrinks and dispels fluid-filled cysts of the breast, ovaries, and testicles. The tea of the dried leaves is used as a substitute for black tea. It has an astringent and mildly alterative effect.

Dosage: According to basic recommendations found under "Dosage of tinctures," pages 49–52 and "Dosage of teas and decoctions," pages 70–71.

External use: As a gargle, 1 or 2 droppersful (30 to 60 drops) of the tincture in ½ cup (120 ml) of water is a useful treatment for sore throat, tonsillitis, and enlarged lymph nodes. A tea of the dried leaves can be used similarly—or just chew a leaf.

Contraindications: Not for use during pregnancy. Do not take red root along with the pharmaceutical anticoagulant warfarin.

Other species: There are 55 species in the *Ceanothus* genus, all woody ground covers, shrubs, or small trees indigenous to North America. Although the eastern species (*C. americanus*) is considered official, one of the western species (*C. velutinas*) is equally strong. Several other western species, including buckbrush (*C. cuneatus*) and deerbrush (*C. integerrimus*), are also used as reasonable substitutes for *C. americanus*.

Rhodiola (Golden Root)
(*Rhodiola rosea*)
Family: Stonecrop (*Crassulaceae*)

Parts used: The spongy, succulent root of plants at least 4 years of age. Highest rosavin content occurs in the late fall after 1 or 2 frosts have descended on the crowns, and again in the spring, just prior to the unfurling of the dormant buds. Some medicinal activity is lost in dehydration, but both fresh herb and dried are serviceable. Wash the roots and slice thinly, then use in the fresh state or shade-dry on screens. These roots are slow to dry, and may take days to snap. Stored in sealed containers in a cool, dry place, the herb maintains its potency for up to 3 years.

Tincture of fresh herb: 1:3 (80A:10W:10GLY) Glycerine stabilizes the tannins. Alcohol is an efficient solvent for the 2 main classes of active constituents: rosavin and salidroside, and so the alcoholic tinctures are probably the most effective way to use the herb. Good quality Rhodiola root will impart an orange-red (almost golden!) color to the finished extract.

Tincture of dry herb: 1:5 (65A:25W:10GLY)

Water extracts: The tea may be made of 4 g of fresh root or 1 g of dried root. Rosavin and salidroside are only grudgingly soluble in hot water. To improve extraction, gently simmer the herb for 10 minutes, then cover and allow to infuse for an additional 10 minutes before drinking.

Rhodiola nastojka: Nastojka is a traditional Russian tincture, in this case a weak alcoholic infusion of Rhodiola root. Use a quart canning jar, pack with fresh or dried root slices, cover generously with brandy or vodka, then screw on the lid and macerate with daily shaking in a warm, dark place for an entire lunar cycle. Then, pour off through cheesecloth and store the orange-red extract in amber glass, tightly stoppered. This is best taken in teaspoonful doses before meals as a tonic and sexual stimulant.

Practical uses: A powerful adaptogen, Rhodiola treats fatigue and exhaustion related to environmental or emotional stress, sleep deprivation, or unaccustomed physical exercise or work. Even a small, once-daily dosage in the morning can help improve mental focus, physical endurance, and productivity. The herb also promotes oxygen uptake and helps one adapt rapidly to high altitude, while reducing symptoms of headache and dizziness. Rhodiola has a gentle yet profound antianxiety effect and may help fight depression and attention deficit disorder (ADD). The herb is also used in weight loss programs, causing rapid oxidation of excess fat and helping control binge eating.

Dosage: Low doses seem to have a more reliable effect than larger doses. Of the tea, 1 to 3 cups daily. Of nastojka, 1 teaspoonful up to 3 times a day before meals. Of the tincture, 5 to 15 drops taken up to 3 times a day.

Contraindications: Generally considered to be safe, nontoxic, and nonaddictive, the herb nonetheless should be taken only according to recommended dosage. Overdose or hypersensitivity can cause symptoms of dry mouth, dizziness, drowsiness, or overstimulation. If the herb causes sleeplessness, take only once per day, in the morning.

Other species: Stonecrops hybridize freely and demonstrate much variation in form within each species. *Rhodiola rosea* is no exception! Circumpolar in distribution, regional variants have been collected from the Alps and the Carpathian Mountains, also from high altitude sites in Russia, Austria, Germany, and throughout Scandinavia. These ecotypes display variation in concentration of active constituents, but are nonetheless effective.

Rhubarb (Chinese Rhubarb, Tibetan Rhubarb, East Indian Rhubarb, or Turkey Rhubarb) (*Rheum palmatum*) Family: Buckwheat (*Polygonaceae*)

Part used: Dried root and crown, without the bark. The roots are harvested during dormancy and the crown split vertically in order to individualize the several taproots. The roots are then washed, the outer bark scraped off with a knife, and the pieces further cut into thick, diagonal sections. These are dried on screens in a warm, dark, and airy place. A forced-air dehydrator is very good for this, or the roots may be strung and spaced apart from each other on a string and suspended over a wood stove, hearth, or other source of dry heat.

Tincture of dried root: 1:5 (50A:40W:10Gly)

Water extract: Basic tea of the dried root. The tea is made with 1 teaspoonful (2 g) of the chopped or ground root, steeped for 15 minutes. The dosage is 1 cup (240 ml) taken before bed.

Syrup: Combine 1 part by volume of the strong decoction:2 parts by volume of honey (see "Chapter 9, Herbal Succi and Syrups").

Practical uses: In small doses, rhubarb is tonic and astringent to the gastrointestinal tract. Large doses are laxative. The herb is used for treating constipation or a feeling of fullness associated with slow transport time. In the case of tropical dysentery, rhubarb assists in the expulsion of the responsible organisms and then tonifies the digestive tract with its gentle astringent action.

Dosage: As with all anthraquinone laxatives, the effects are delayed for several hours. For astringent and tonic activity, take ½ dropperful of the tincture or a teaspoon of the syrup twice daily. For laxative effect, the normal adult dosage is 2 droppersful (60 drops) of the tincture or 4 tablespoons (20 ml) of the syrup in warm water just prior to bed. This assures an efficient movement first thing in the morning.

Contraindications: Not to be taken during pregnancy. Not to be taken while nursing (laxative effects go through the milk). Not to be taken by children. Do not take if there is intestinal obstruction. Long-term usage may result in dependency.

Other species: The historical search for the plant responsible for the "official" laxative rhubarb root of world commerce makes a good story. Although this popular item was sold in the bazaars of Turkey (therefore the misnomer "Turkey rhubarb"), the actual origin proved to be China. It took early traders and explorers a long, long time to discover this secret, and even longer to carry the verified seeds of this plant back to Europe. Turkey rhubarb (*Rheum palmatum*) produces a beautiful, palmate leaf and a fleshy root that is richly endowed with the laxative, yellow-colored anthraquinones. Other species which are used interchangeably for the laxative and astringent effects are Himalayan rhubarb (*R. emodi*) and another herb that is commonly called Chinese rhubarb (*R. officinale*). Garden rhubarb (*R. rhabarbarum, R. hybridum,* or *R. rhaponticum*) looks similar to these, but is appreciated more for the red stems, sugared and used in pies, since these plants contain very minimal quantities of the laxative anthraquinones.

Flaxseed (linseed) *(Linum usitatissimum)* **as a substitute for anthraquinone laxatives:** By the way, 1 tablespoonful ground flaxseed taken internally with plenty of water, morning and night, is emollient to the gastric lining and promotes regular and comfortable bowel movements. Flaxseed is not habit-forming.

Rosemary, Official (*Rosmarinus officinalis*)
Family: Mint (*Lamiaceae*)

Parts used: Leaf and flowers stripped from the branches and used fresh or dried.

Tincture of fresh herb: 1:2 (100A)

Tincture of dried herb: 1:5 (75A:25W)

Water extracts: Basic tea of fresh or dried herb.

Direct consumption: Chew a few of the fresh leaves.

Practical uses: Legion. Rosemary is a classic digestive, nerve, and circulatory tonic. It is a good treatment for low energy, low blood pressure, and poor circulation. The herb improves memory, gives courage, and lifts the spirits.

Dosage: According to basic recommendations found under "Dosage of tinctures," pages 49–52 and "Dosage of teas and decoctions," pages 70–71.

External use: The tincture, tea, or even the fresh plant may be rubbed freely into areas of poor circulation. To gently stimulate a weak heart, rub into the heart region of chest. A rosemary bath is an excellent diaphoretic and circulation stimulant (see page 100). To discourage lice infestation, the essential oil or strong tincture can be used for dressing the hair and hairbrush.

Food use: Rosemary has long been employed as a spice for oily fish and poultry, imparting its characteristic aroma even if over-cooked. The herb is an effective preservative and antioxidant, extending shelf-life of stored foods and in the human body, limiting the incidence of cellular damage that can be attributed to eating saturated fats cooked at high temperature.

Contraindications: Food use during pregnancy is fine. Avoid direct contact with pure, undiluted essential oil of rosemary on sensitive skin.

Other species: There are more than 25 cultivars of rosemary, offering an array of sizes and differing somewhat in aroma and chemistry. Standard upright types tend to be the best for spice and medicinal use.

Sage, Garden (*Salvia officinalis*)
Family: Mint (*Lamiaceae*)

Parts used: Leaves harvested from plants just prior to flowering, in the afternoon of a bright day, stripped from the stem and used fresh or dried.

Tincture of fresh herb: 1:2 (100A)

Tincture of dried herb: 1:5 (75A:25W)

Water extract: Basic tea of the dried herb.

Practical uses: Garden sage is a valuable antibacterial, antifungal, and antiviral agent. Taken internally, the herb will fight infection and will also diminish secretions of all kinds, including perspiration and saliva. Garden sage tea or tincture is a specific for drying up milk production during weaning. The herb stimulates memory.

Dosage: According to basic recommendations found under "Dosage of tinctures," pages 49–52 and "Dosage of teas and decoctions," pages 70–71.

External: Sage makes an antibacterial mouthwash and astringent gargle for treating sore throat. Use the tea, or dilute the tincture at the rate of 1 dropperful (30 drops) per ½ cup (120 ml) of water.

Food use: Sage is an agreeable spice if not used in excess, a requisite ingredient for making stuffing for roasted poultry, and sometimes used for seasoning meats and other protein dishes.

Contraindications: Not for use during pregnancy, except as a culinary spice. Sage contains thujone, which in excessive quantity is potentially toxic. Do not exceed recommended dosage, and do not take at medicinal dosage on an ongoing basis. Avoid direct contact with pure, undiluted essential oil of sage, especially on sensitive skin, mucous membranes, and in the eyes.

Other species: Although garden sage is official, the 750 other species belonging to the genus *Salvia* are also largely used in medicine. These plants present far too much variability to allow for generalization about their medicinal effects. This becomes apparent simply by sniffing the completely different aromas produced by, for instance white sage (*S. apiana*), Middle-Eastern sage (*S. fruticosa*), and Chinese red sage (dan-shen) (*S. miltiorrhiza*). These are all employed in their native lands as medicinals, but for different purposes. The genus ranges from the practically inodorous species blue sage (*S. azurea*) to the most potent of all sage flowers, borne by clary sage (*S. sclarea*), dubbed by my children "the armpit plant." In aromatherapy, this one is said to carry the scent of erotica. The flowers do smell, that's for sure, but the leaves of clary sage have practically no smell. Then, the leaves of Dominican sage (*S. dominica*) smell like the flowers of clary sage, but only when fresh, and once dried, smell completely different again. Given that these various aromas are linked to the degree and kind of biological activity, you are now getting an idea of the diversity of the medicinal attributes of the *Salvias*. The genus is similarly diverse in terms of growth habit, ranging from annuals such as scarlet sage (*S. coccinea*) to biennials like clary sage (*S. sclarea*), to woody perennials such as white sage (*S. apiana*) and black sage (*S. mellifera*).

Saint John's Wort (*Hypericum perforatum*)
Family: Saint John's Wort (*Hypericaceae*)

Parts used: Flowering and budding tops, consisting of approximately the top 10 inches (25 cm) of the plant and used fresh or dried. The fresh flowering tops are usually processed along with the associated stems. The dried herb may be rubbed through a screen, thereby separating out the stems, which can be composted. Whether using the herb in the fresh or dry state, resist the temptation to use only the flowers. The leaf contains active flavonoids, which augment the activity of the compounds (hypericins) found in the flowers and buds.

Tincture of fresh herb: 1:2 (100A)

Tincture of recently dried herb: 1:5 (75A:25W)
Contrary to general belief, making tincture with dried, rather than fresh, Saint John's wort is an extremely effective preparation.[15]

Water extract: Basic tea of the dried herb.

Practical uses: Saint John's wort has a deep-seated nervine effect, helping restore damaged nerve tissue, deadening nerve pain (including sciatica), and strengthening the urinary organs. The herb is very useful for treating athletic injuries with nerve damage and/or pulled muscles or ligaments, also for improving quality of life for those suffering from chronic disease, including arthritis, multiple sclerosis, and AIDS. "Hypericum," which translates literally as "over an apparition" is a proven antidepressant that definitely helps raise the spirits.

Dosage: According to basic recommendations found under "Dosage of tinctures," pages 49–52 and "Dosage of teas and decoctions," pages 70–71.

Oil infusion of fresh flowering and budding tops only: Combine 1 part by weight of the fresh herb:3 parts by volume of olive oil. The dried herb does not extract in oil. The fresh herb should be thoroughly bruised or mashed prior to combining with the oil. The flower stems serve the function of allowing oil flow around the mashed flowers and leaves, which otherwise tend to clump. Follow the basic procedure for making fresh herb infused oils (see page 83). Solar maceration of the oily extract improves extraction of certain constituents, although maceration in the dark is also effective. The maceration must be continued for 2 full weeks. This "hypericated oil" is a useful external application for bruises, sprains, swellings, varicose ulcers, hemorrhoids, and old burns (see page 99). The oil may be further processed into salve or cream, which retains the same effect (see pages 85–90). The oil can also be used internally as a treatment for indigestion and/or gastric ulcer. The internal dosage is 1 teaspoon (5 ml) taken 2 to 3 times daily. See "Contraindications."

---

[15]The tincture of good quality dried leaves and flowers attains a deep burgundy-red and tastes like the herb smells on a hot day in a high meadow. The sometimes-recommended practice of macerating the *alcoholic* extract in the sun (solar maceration), however, does not increase content of the hypericins and actually produces an inferior tincture.

Contraindications: Not to be taken concurrently with pharmaceutical drugs. Do not exceed recommended dosage. Overdose of the herb can cause photosensitivity, generally characterized by an increased optical sensitivity to sunlight and an increased tendency for the sun to burn the skin. People with fair complexions should be especially cautious not to overdose on this herb. Areas treated with the infused oil of Saint John's wort should be kept covered from the sun, due to an increased risk of burning or blistering and the rare incidence of permanent darkening of skin pigmentation resulting from solar exposure after applying the oil.

Harvesting and processing cautions: Take care during harvest and handling of the fresh herb, because hypericins are readily absorbed through the skin. Using gloves is recommended. Following handling of large quantities of fresh herb, make sure that all exposed skin surfaces are thoroughly washed with soap and water. While harvesting in the hot sun, take care not to wipe the delicate tissues around the eyes or the brow with hypericin-laden hands. These areas are particularly sensitive.

Other species: There are 300 species in the *Hypericum* genus found worldwide. None of them live up to true Saint John's wort in terms of overall medicinal functionality. Western St. John's wort (*H. formosum*) contains only a small amount of hypericin. It is readily confused with *H. perforatum.* Western St. John's wort is a diminutive plant with a stem that is round in cross-section, not grooved like the stem of our Saint John's wort. This plant is native to the west coast of North America, from Britsh Columbia to California and inland as far as Montana and Wyoming.

Savory, Summer (*Satureja hortensis*)
Family: Mint (*Lamiaceae*)

Part used: The leaves and small stems, either fresh or dried. Harvest prior to flowering, in the afternoon of a warm day, by cutting the top half of the plant off with shears. The bottom half of the plant is left behind in order to support growth of a new crop of succulent tops, as up to 3 cuttings may be made in a season. Also, the lower leaves are less choice because they are often splashed with dirt and sand, while the more aerial parts of the plant remain quite clean. Dry on screens or by bundling and hanging in a warm room with good air flow. Once the stems snap when bent, rub the herb through a ⅛ inch screen, allowing the dried leaf to accrue on a clean tabletop. The stems will remain on top of the screen, and may be composted or used as an aromatic fire starter. The dried herb may be screened once again to remove more stem, then stored in sealed containers in a cool, dark place, retaining its goodness for at least 1 year.

Tincture of fresh herb: 1:2 (90A:10GLY) Glycerin is added in order to stabilize the tannins.

Tincture of dried herb: 1:5 (70A:20W:10GLY)

Acetum of dried herb: 1:7 (100ACV); see page 55.

Acetum of fresh herb: Pack the fresh, preflowering tops in a quart jar right up to the shoulder and then cover generously with apple cider vinegar. Keep on the windowsill in the sun for a week, with daily shaking. Then, strain out the fresh herb and store the herbal vinegar in amber glass. This is an excellent base for salad dressings, lending a delicious taste and preserving oils against oxidation in storage.

Oil, salve, or cream: Make infused herbal oil of the dried herb. This can be used as-is or may be further processed into salve or cream (see "Chapter 10, Basic Formulas for Herbal Oils, Salves, and Creams," pages 85–90). Oily extractions of summer savory have a warming effect on the skin and have traditionally been used as massage oils. The effect is stimulating to the circulation. Rubbed on the lower back and back of legs, the oil helps prevent cramping and sciatica.

Poultice: Smash the fresh, juicy tops and apply to beesting for immediate relief of pain and swelling. One of the best ways to do this is the "mouth poultice." Chew the herb and apply wet.

Water extract: Basic tea of dried leaves.

Practical uses: Savory, true to its name, is among the tastiest of all culinary/medicinal herbs. Therefore, it may be added to multi-ingredient tinctures as a flavoring agent and preservative. The tea or diluted tincture may be gargled to treat sore throat.

The effect is astringent and pain-relieving, due to the presence of astringent tannins and antiseptic compounds including thymol and carvacrol. The preservative and anxiolytic (calming and antidepressant) effects of summer savory are attributable in part to the presence of rosmarinic acid. Rosmarinic acid content varies depending on harvest time, with the highest levels present during the hottest month of the year.

Dosage: According to basic recommendations found under "Dosage of tinctures," pages 49–52, "Dosage of dried herb aceta, pages 55–56," and "Dosage of teas and decoctions," pages 70–71.

Food use: As a culinary spice, the fresh or dried savory leaf is added to food near the end of preparation, in order to prevent the tasty and aromatic essential oils from volatilizing. The antioxidant properties help prevent cellular damage from ingestion of fats and oils, so the herb is commonly added to the flour used to dredge poultry prior to frying. Used as a spice, savory is peppery in taste, and is perhaps the quintessential carminative, warming the fires of digestion and eliminating gas. For this reason, it is often used in bean dishes, although in my home at least, as my relations will attest, it is used in almost *every* dish!

Contraindications: Summer savory is safe for general use. Do not take the pure essential oil of savory internally. Avoid direct contact with pure, undiluted essential oil of savory, especially on sensitive skin, mucous membranes, and in eyes.

Other species: *Satureja* is a wide-ranging genus with its gene center in the Mediterranean basin. Wherever savory grows, it finds its way into local cuisine and medicine. Winter savory (*Satureja montana*) contains lower concentrations of essential oil than summer savory, and the mounding, bush-like foliage is less kind to the touch, but it is a reasonable substitute nonetheless. Unlike summer savory, this one is available in the fresh state all winter long! Savory of Crete (*Satureja thymbra*) is a dominant subshrub on the Island of Crete, where it is employed by the inhabitants as a culinary spice. The essential oil of savory of Crete is quite famous. Diluted in a carrier oil and used in massage, essential oil of savory of Crete exerts a pain-relieving and relaxing influence. This is one of the best savories worldwide.

Schisandra (Wu-wei-zi) (*Schizandra chinensis*)
Family: Magnolia (*Magnoliaceae*)

Part used: Ripe berries used fresh or dried.

Tincture of fresh berries: 1:2 (100A)
The berries are mashed or blended in the menstruum.

Tincture of dried berries (very strong): 1:4 (75A:25W)
The berries are soaked overnight, blended in the menstruum, then macerated in the usual manner.

Water extract: Cold infusion or basic tea of dried berries.

Practical uses: Schisandra is a nutritive and immune-enhancing tonic. The herb is good for treating cough, shortness of breath, impotency, stress, tiredness, allergies, chronic gastritis, and dysentery. Schisandra stimulates salivation and gastric secretion.

Dosage: According to basic recommendations found under "Dosage of tinctures," pages 49–52 and "Dosage of teas and decoctions," pages 70–71.

Contraindications: None known. Safe for general use.

Self-Heal (*Prunella vulgaris*)
Family: Mint (*Lamiaceae*)

Parts used: Mature flower heads picked after the morning dew has evaporated and used fresh or dried. Stems and leaves may also be used.

Tincture of dried herb: 1:5 (50A:40W:10Gly)

Tincture of fresh herb: 1:2 (65A:25W:10Gly)

Water extracts: Basic tea or decoction of the fresh or dried herb.

Syrup: Make a strong decoction of the dried herb and combine 1:2 with honey. Follow procedure found in "Chapter 9, Herbal Succi and Syrups."

Practical uses: Self-heal is one of the most useful of healing astringents, and is a specific for treating herpes lesions of the mucous membranes. It can be taken internally as a tea, tincture, or syrup for a general tonic effect.

External use: As a wash for wounds or as a gargle for treating sore throat, use the water extract full-strength or dilute 1 dropperful (30 drops) of the tincture in ½ cup (120 ml) of cold water. For direct application to canker sores, use the water extract or tincture full-strength—swish and spit. Effective for treating oral lesions (herpes type 1) and genital lesions (herpes type 2). The herb deadens pain and speeds resolution of the problem. Concurrent internal use of the herb can be of assistance.

Dosage: According to basic recommendations found under "Dosage of tinctures," pages 49–52 and "Dosage of teas and decoctions," pages 70–71.

Contraindications: None known. Safe for general use.

Shepherd's Purse (*Capsella bursa-pastoris*) Family: Mustard (*Brassicaceae*)

Parts used: Entire fresh plant, with root, in flower.

Tincture of fresh herb: 1:1.5 (75A:25W) Blender method, p. 22. Cut the stemmy herb and root into short pieces with scissors before blending. The tincture remains viable for only 1 year.

Practical uses: Shepherd's purse is a vasoconstrictor with an affinity for the smooth muscles of the uterus and gastrointestinal tract. Taken internally, it is used primarily to arrest heavy menses (menorrhagia) and to stop diarrhea. The tincture may also be applied externally on a cloth, used to staunch blood from wounds or bloody nose. The herb also has an oxytocic effect, used to augment contractions during active labor (4 to 7 cm dilation), to control postpartum hemorrhage, to tonify the uterus, and help prevent prolapse. There are several drawbacks. First off, the tincture has a short shelf-life and tastes terrible—like broccoli soup forgotten for days at the back of the kitchen counter. Combining with rosemary (70% shepherd's purse to 30% rosemary by volume) may help prolong the shelf-life and mask the taste. Secondly, the herb doesn't always work. Some women report good results in controlling menorrhagia, while others experience no relief. Successful treatment with shepherd's purse may be dosage-dependent, and if a little tincture fails to do the job, it will not hurt to try larger and more frequent doses.

Dosage: To tonify the uterus, arrest heavy menses, or treat diarrhea, take 10 to 20 drops up to 5 times a day. During active labor, 30 drops of the tincture may be taken every 5 minutes until the baby is born.

Contraindications: Although shepherd's purse is safe to take during active labor, it is not a good idea to take it during pregnancy, as the herb stimulates contractions. Heavy bleeding may be a sign of miscarriage, uterine fibroids, polyps, or other serious conditions. Seek the assistance of a qualified health care practitioner.

Skullcap (*Scutellaria lateriflora*)
Family: Mint (*Lamiaceae*)

Parts used: Entire aerial portions of the plant, including stems, leaves, and flowers, used fresh or dried.

Tincture of fresh plant (preferred): 1:2 (75A:25W); see page 42.

Tincture of dried plant: 1:5 (50A:50W)

Water extract: Basic tea of fresh or dried herb.

Succus of fresh herb: 1 part alcohol by volume: 3 parts skullcap juice by volume (see "Chapter 9, Herbal Succi and Syrups").

Practical uses: Skullcap is a nervine tonic, sedative, and antispasmodic. The herb is useful in treating nervous agitation, hysteria, anxiety, insomnia, nerve pain, and tremors.

Dosage: Starting adult dosage of the tincture is 1 dropperful (30 drops) taken 2 to 3 times daily, more or less depending on body size, sensitivity, and severity of the problem.

Contraindications: Do not exceed recommended dosage. Side effects resulting from overdose or oversensitivity may include dizziness, giddiness, confusion, or loss of concentration. If any of these symptoms arise, reduce dosage or discontinue use.

Other species: There are about 300 species of the *Scutellaria* genus occurring worldwide. Although *S. lateriflora* (sometimes

264

erroneously adaged *S. laterifolia*) is generally accepted as the "official" species, local herbalists will use local species like marsh skullcap (*S. galericulata)* and heart-leaved skullcap (*S. versicolor*) with good results. Baical skullcap (*S. baicalensis*) has its own set of indications, really quite different from the nervine skullcaps, and cannot be used interchangeably with them.

Slippery Elm (*Ulmus rubra*)
Family: Elm (*Ulmaceae*)

Parts used: The inner bark (the bast or phloem), harvested in the spring when the sap is up. Fall-harvested bast is more astringent and therefore less desirable than the spring-harvested material. As long as the tree is healthy, the older the tree, the better, as older trees produce a thicker and juicier inner bark. Cut the lowest branch of the tree off right at the trunk. Make a shallow undercut first, to keep the branch from stripping off the bark of the trunk when it falls. Watch out when it falls—stand clear. Using its own mucilage, the tree will soon seal off the wound, and will not ultimately be harmed by this practice. Using a drawknife, ross the rough exterior bark off of the branch, down to the beige inner bark. Once the outer bark is removed, go over the branch once again with the draw knife, but this time remove the bast in long strips, right down to the wood, which will be slippery with sap. Collect the bast strips and cut them up into 6-inch pieces right away, while still moist. Lay the pieces out on screens in the sun, turning once or twice daily, and cover at night so the dew does not rewet them. Thus handled, the pieces will dry in 2 to 3 days. Use the pieces as-is to make the cold infusion, or grind them down to a powder, in which form the herb truly has a myriad of uses. Store in sealed jars, out of the light.

Water extracts: Since alcohol precipitates the mucilage, the tincture is not recommended. The best preparation is the cold infusion, made by putting a piece of the dried inner bark (weighing between 7 and 10 g) in a large glass (500 ml) of water and infuse overnight. In the morning, remove the bark from the mucilage-laden water and slurp a little at a time, throughout the day. A little slippery elm goes a long way! See page 68.

Powdered slippery elm is quick and efficient for making a mucilage-laden drink. Use 1 heaping teaspoonful (5 g) in 1 pint (473 ml) of cold water. To avoid clumping, sift the powder slowly into the water and keep whisking with a chopstick or fork until the powder is smoothly incorporated. To make a hot tea, it is best to sift the powder into the cold water and stir vigorously, then slowly bring the tea to a simmer before pouring into a cup and drinking. Alternatively, make a paste of a little water and slippery elm powder, then introduce the paste to the larger volume of liquid, stir vigorously to incorporate, and then simmer before pouring into a cup and drinking.

Practical uses: The hot tea is best for treating sore throat, coughs, or bronchitis, whether caused by upper respiratory infection or excessive use (ministering to the flock, belting raucous rock). In any case, the tea will soothe and heal. The cold infusion is best for treating inflammation of the stomach, small intestine or colon. Slippery elm is harmless, and may be used to treat simple upset stomach or stomach cramps, but also works very well for treating infant colic, dysentery, stomach or duodenal ulcers, diverticulitis, and inflammatory bowel disease (IBD), including ulcerative colitis and Crohn's disease. The mucilage soothes and replenishes mucous membranes, absorbs toxins, moves them out of the body, and nourishes the mast cells that reside at the foundations of our immunity.

Direct consumption: The fresh or dried bast may be chewed to slowly release its healing mucilage. One need not be sick to enjoy the nourishment and soothing grace of the chaw that keeps on giving. A premier survival food or trailside snack.

Poultice: Put slippery elm powder in a shallow bowl and, stirring briskly, add sufficient hot water to make a thick goo and spread this immediately on 2 layers of cheesecloth, up to ½ inch thick. Transfer the cheesecloth to the affected area, then cover with moist, hot towels to insulate. This is an excellent treatment for swollen glands, infections, splinters, eruptions, and wounds. This poultice also works well as a carrier for other medicinal herbs. When treating infections, stir in a dropperful of goldenseal tincture. To speed healing, stir in a dropperful of comfrey or

266

calendula tincture. To treat burns, make the poultice with cold water. Poultices are best kept on for at least 20 minutes, overnight if possible.

Gruel: In a double boiler or in a saucepan on low flame, begin to heat up 3 cups of water or milk (dairy or nut derived). Sift in 1½ tablespoons of slippery elm powder while whisking vigorously to incorporate. Continue to heat and occasionally stir the gruel until it thickens, then remove from heat and sweeten with honey or maple syrup before serving. This is herbal food, a nutritious breakfast that may be enjoyed by anyone. Hungry people, infants suffering the ravages of teething, elders with weak stomachs, patients recuperating from surgery or suffering from wasting diseases will be nourished and uplifted.

Contraindications: Safe for general use.

Other species: All species of *Ulmus* will yield a bit of mucilage from the bast, but none compare to *Ulmus rubra*—the very best.

Small-Flowered-Willow-Herb (*Epilobium parviflorum*) Family: Evening Primrose (*Onagraceae*)

Parts used: Fresh or dried aerial portions of the plant, including stem, leaf, and flowers, collected prior to seeding.

Tincture of fresh herb: 1:2 (75A:15W:10Gly)

Tincture of dried herb: 1:5 (50A:40W:10Gly)

Water extracts: The basic tea of the dried herb is preferred. Basic tea of fresh herb. Decoction of dried herb.

Direct consumption: The herb is an edible green.

Practical uses: Small-flowered-willow-herb is an astringent and diuretic, used to help detoxify the urinary tract. It is a specific for treating benign prostatitis, where there is a proliferation of cells causing swelling, urinary dysfunction, and eventually pain. The herb helps shrink the tissues, arrest cell proliferation, normalize urinary function, and prevent onset of more serious disorders.

Dosage: According to basic recommendations found under "Dosage of tinctures," pages 49–52 and "Dosage of teas and decoctions," pages 70–71.

Poultice: The fresh, bruised or mashed plant, including the root, makes a cooling poultice, which will help in healing of wounds, ulcerations, and old burns.

Contraindications: None known. Safe for general use.

Other species: The *Epilobium* genus is represented by over 200 species widely distributed throughout the temperate north. The most conspicuous of these is fireweed (*E. angustifolium*), which is used as a substitute for black tea, as an edible green, and, like *E. parviflorum,* as a treatment for prostatitis. Fireweed herb is very high in tannins, as well as active flavonoids. It has been used traditionally as an anti-inflammatory poultice, and taken internally as a tea to stem diarrhea. Local herbalists are also using it as a treatment for candidiasis. Other species of willow-herb that can be used interchangeably with *E. parviflorum* and *E. angustifolium* are *E. montanum, E. roseum,* and *E. collinum.*

Sorrel, Sheep (*Rumex acetosella*)
Family: Buckwheat (*Polygonaceae*)

Parts used: The entire plant harvested prior to flowering, including the root. This is an herb of spring, and may be found growing luxuriously in loose, moist soils or sand. Sheep sorrel is an enthusiastic spreader, and a single individual can easily become a large patch. I always wondered why, when seed collecting, I would find some patches to be entirely seedless and others to be full of seeds. Then, I learned that the plant is dioecious (having both male plants and female plants), and realized that in all likelihood the seedless patch was composed entirely of one male plant, and that the seeded patch was actually composed of only one female plant! The underground system of creeping rhizomes (the root) was thus shown to be substantial. Given that the tannin-rich root is one of the most valuable parts of the plant for making medicine, care should be taken during harvest to get as much root as possible. Carefully wash the threadlike, elastic roots to remove soil particles, then cut into pieces with scissors and process in the blender or dry on screens for future use. Drying (as well as cooking) reduces the load of oxalic acid. Store in sealed containers in a cool, dark place. The dried herb remains viable for only 1 year.

Tincture of fresh herb: 1:2 (75A:15W:10Gly)

Tincture of dried herb: 1:5 (50A:40W:10Gly)

Water extracts: The basic tea or decoction of the dried herb is preferred over trying to make the tea from fresh herb. Sheep sorrel is also used in tea formulas. According to popular belief, this is the most essential anticancer ingredient in "Essiac tea."

Direct consumption: Children have a way of letting each other know about common edible plants, and sheep sorrel is a case in point. The sweet-tart flavor of the fresh leaves really attracts them! Of course, this taste is also an indication of oxalic acid content, so it is good to advise children to chew in moderation. As an occasional salad ingredient, the arrowhead-shaped leaves lend a vinegary taste. In creamy soups, incorporating a little of the fresh herb imparts an agreeable tartness. It boils right down.

Practical uses: Sheep sorrel is most commonly employed to fight degenerative diseases including runaway bacterial infection, parasitic infestations, and cancer. The herb is powerfully astringent, exerting a deep-seated effect on body tissues and organs—detoxification and tonification. Sheep sorrel is antineoplastic, inhibiting proliferation of abnormal cells while ridding the body of endotoxins and other metabolic waste. The plant is loaded with bioavailable vitamins, trace minerals, and tannins that help promote regrowth of healthy tissue.

Dosage: According to basic recommendations found under "Dosage of tinctures," pages 49–52 and "Dosage of teas and decoctions," pages 70–71.

Contraindications: Large doses or daily use should be avoided, due to high oxalic acid content. Sheep sorrel should not be used during pregnancy or nursing, or if suffering from arthritis, rheumatism, gout, or kidney stones. Calcium oxalate is the most common component of kidney stones.

Other species: The family *Polygonaceae* represents about 1,200 species, including a large number of powerfully active medicinal plants. Turkey rhubarb (*Rheum palmatum*) is one of them, an anthraquinone laxative of great renown. Like sheep sorrel, Turkey rhubarb is an ingredient in the Essiac formula, and also contains oxalic acid. Yellow dock (*Rumex crispus*) is similar to both of the above herbs, an alterative that is full of minerals, especially iron, that also exerts a laxative influence. Japanese knotweed (*Polygonum cuspicatum*), like sheep sorrel spreads enthusiastically. The root of this plant contains resveratrol, a polyphenolic compound that inhibits tumors and helps prolong life through the telomeric effect—protecting the ends of the human chromosome from age-related deterioration.

Spikenard (*Aralia californica, A. racemosa*)
Family: Ginseng (*Araliaceae*)

Parts used: Root and rhizome (the root) dug in dormancy. The leaves and berries harvested at maturity and used fresh or dried.

Tincture of fresh root or fresh berries: 1:2 (75A:25W)

Tincture of recently dried root or dried berries: 1:5 (50A:50W)

Water extracts: Basic tea of fresh or dried leaves, with or without the berries. Decoction of fresh or recently dried root.

Syrup: Combine 1 part by volume of the strong decoction:2 parts by volume of honey. For general directions on making syrups and a special recipe for compound syrup of spikenard, see "Chapter 9, Herbal Succi and Syrups," pages 77–78.

Direct consumption: A small piece of the leaf, fresh root, or a few fresh berries may be slowly chewed or held in the mouth for their fortifying and expectorant action. A little bit goes a long way, as the fresh, unprocessed plant material can be mildly acrid, in a ginseng sort of a way.

Practical uses: Spikenard has an adaptogenic influence, strengthening the entire system against stress, with a definite affinity for the upper respiratory, digestive, and reproductive organs. The herb is a good expectorant, antimicrobial, and antitussive for treating upper respiratory infection. Consistent with the Native American use, spikenard may be given safely during difficult labor to provide much-needed energy to mother and baby; for this purpose, combines well with blue cohosh.

Dosage: According to basic recommendations found under "Dosage of tinctures," pages 49–52 and "Dosage of teas and decoctions," pages 70–71. Also see basic adult dosage for compound syrup of spikenard, page 78.

Poultice: The fresh root may be pounded and applied to bruises, swellings, splinters, pustules, or rheumatic joints. The poultice has a drawing, cleansing, and anti-inflammatory influence.

Contraindications: Do not exceed recommended dosage. Undiluted spikenard extracts or direct consumption of the plant may irritate mucous membranes of mouth and throat.

Other species: Several prodigious herbs of the *Araliaceae* family are closely allied in their adaptogenic and blood-cleansing activity. These include spikenard, devil's club (*Oplopanax horridum*), eleuthero (*Eleutherococcus senticosus*), American ginseng (*Panax quinquefolius*), and wild sarsaparilla (*Aralia nudicaulis*). The two true spikenards (*Aralia californica and A. racemosa*) are medicinally interchangeable and bear the distinction of being the largest of the North American *Araliaceae* as well as being the easiest to cultivate. See "Eleuthero" and "Ginseng, American."

Spilanthes (*Acmella oleracea, A. alba*)
Family: Aster (*Asteraceae*)

Parts used: Entire plant, including root, stem, leaf, and especially the young flower buds and flowers, harvested in full flower and used either fresh or dried.

Tincture of fresh herb: 1:2 (100A)

Tincture of recently dried herb: 1:5 (75A:25W)

Direct consumption: The fresh leaves or buds, taken as needed and held in the mouth, and eventually ingested. The dried buds are less of a tactile treat, but still deliver the essence of the plant.

271

Practical uses: Spilanthes has an immune-enhancing effect, which is of utility in the case of beginning-phase infections, both viral and bacterial, including children's earaches, impetigo, and thrush. The herb strongly promotes salivation, for treating dryness of mouth and poor appetite, is stimulating to both the lymphatic system and the general circulation, and acts as an oral antiseptic for treating various dental woes, including swelling, gum disease, decay, and mouth sores, such as canker sores, herpes, and cold sores; swish after brushing. Spilanthes is pro-phylactic and curative for blood parasites, including malarial spirochetes, and is of assistance in treating Lyme disease. The herb strongly inhibits the yeast organism *Candida albicans*, which is responsible for the condition known as candidiasis. Use of spilanthes is a valuable adjunct therapy in treating diseases caused by drug-resistant bacteria and viruses.

Dosage: According to basic recommendations found under "Dosage of tinctures," pages 49–52. The plant synergizes well with echinacea. To treat an acute infection such as an child's earache, a program that is usually effective is to alternate 6 to 8 drop dosages first of spilanthes, then of echinacea, every ½ hour until the infection abates.

Food use: Spilanthes leaves are used sparingly in salad and soup.

Contraindications: Daily internal use or daily chewing of the leaves or flowering buds in season may reduce the entire load of intestinal bacteria, both pathogenic and probiotic. Therefore, continuous internal use of the herb is not recommended. Spilanthes may be used as a mouthwash several times a day without any adverse effects.

Other species: There are at least 13 closely-related types found worldwide and although the ethnographic record of native uses is a bit scanty, they are, on the whole, used everywhere to treat the same conditions and are apparently equally harmless. Further investigation into the taxonomic and medicinal attributes of Spilanthes is well-warranted. The conservation and proliferation of each strain of these ancient plants is much needed.

Stevia (*Stevia rebaudiana*)
Family: Aster (*Asteraceae*)

Parts used: Leaves and succulent stems harvested just prior to flowering and used fresh or dried.

Tincture of fresh herb: 1:2 (75A:25W)

Tincture of dried herb: 1:5 (50A:50W)

Glycerite of fresh herb: 1:2 (100Gly)

Water extracts: Basic tea or decoction of fresh or dried herb. Small quantities of the dried herb are added to other tea ingredients as a sweetener.

Practical uses: Stevia is a nonsugar sweetening agent and flavoring for ordinary drinks or for medicinal teas. The dried herb is said to be 250 times sweeter than white sugar. The herb may be used to normalize hypoglycemia, as a sweetener for use by diabetics, as a digestive aid, and as an astringent wound-healer.

Dosage: To sweeten a cup of tea, add 2 to 5 drops of stevia tincture or glycerite. The quantity used is best determined by individual taste.

Contraindications: The herb is not appropriate for flavoring bitters. Stevia is purportedly safe for use by diabetics, but this should nonetheless be approached with circumspection.

Stoneroot (*Collinsonia canadensis*)
Family: Mint (*Lamiaceae*)

Part used: Rhizome (the root) harvested during dormancy and used fresh or dried. The entire plant, including root, nonwoody stems, leaves, and flowers, harvested in full flower and used fresh or dried. The fresh root is difficult to reduce into suitable-sized particles for tincturing. It can be run through a hammer mill, snipped with heavy shears, or smashed with a hammer. If the root is to be dried and stored for later use, it needs to be ground, snipped, or smashed into small pieces while fresh and then dried, because once dry, it is intractable and as hard as bone.

Tincture of fresh herb (preferred): 1:2 (75A:25W). Due to the hardness of the root, stoneroot tinctures are macerated with daily agitation for a period of at least 5 weeks in order to accomplish complete extraction.

Tincture of dried herb: 1:5 (50A:50W)

Water extract: Decoction of the fresh or dried root.

Practical uses: Stoneroot is astringent and tonic to the vascular system and mucous membranes. The herb is appropriately used for treating varicose veins, spider veins, and hemorrhoids. Stoneroot is also a useful treatment for inflammation of the kidneys and bladder. The herb is a specific for "minister's sore throat," a bogginess of tissues of the larynx, caused by over-zealous use of voice.

Dosage: According to basic recommendations found under "Dosage of tinctures," pages 49–52 and "Dosage of teas and decoctions," pages 70–71.

External use: Stoneroot is considered a specific for treating hoarseness and laryngitis. A gargle consisting of the full-strength decoction or 1 dropperful (30 drops) of the tincture diluted in ½ cup (120 ml) of cold water is recommended.

Poultice: The fresh leaves are bruised or mashed and laid on varicosities, swellings, or ulcerations for the astringent and healing effects. They are smooth and cooling.

Contraindications: Safe for general use.

Processing cautions: When smashing fresh stoneroot with a hammer, wear protective goggles.

𝒥

Tea (*Camellia sinensis*)
Family: Tea (*Theaceae*)

Part used: The leaves, especially the tender, immature sprigs. To make green tea, the leaves are cured and roasted. To make black tea, the leaves are cured and roasted, then fermented and dried.

Water extract: Basic tea (a little joke).

Practical uses: Tea is stimulating to the nervous system, generally taken as a congenial beverage, and useful in dispelling certain kinds of headache. Green tea (and to a lesser extent black tea) is a concentrated source of the phenolic compounds known as catechins, which are potent cell protectors, guarding against carcinonogenesis and slowing the growth of cancerous tumors.

External use: Tea is a valuable astringent for treating skin eruptions and allergic reactions or inflammations. The strong infusion can be used directly as a wash. Tea also makes a very effective astringent and pain-relieving sitz bath for treating hemorrhoids.

Contraindications: Taken in excess, tea can cause nervous excitability and sleeplessness.

Other species: There are approximately 80 species in the *Camellia* genus found worldwide. *C. sinensis* is the official tea plant, which can be successfully grown in the highland tropics as well as in California and in the southern states of North America. This plant has been selected, over time, into numerous regional cultivars. The differences in taste perceived among teas from different growing areas can be attributed as much to climate, cultivation practices, harvesting, and post-harvest processing as to varietal characteristics. *Camellia japonica* is the main decorative species in this genus, consisting of over 3,000 named varieties. These are beautiful in the garden, but are not much used in medicine.

Tea Tree (*Melaleuca alternifolia*)
Family: Myrtle (*Myrtaceae*)

Part used: The leaves, separated from the woody branches and used fresh or dried. Tea tree oil is an essential oil obtained from trees grown in subtropical areas. The trees are generally cut right back down to a stump, which coppices (resprouts) and eventually provides another cutting, and then another. In temperate climates, the trees may be kept in pots or planted in the greenhouse and the leaves harvested in the fall by pruning the branches.

Tincture of the fresh leaf: 1:2 (100A)

Tincture of the dried leaf: 1:5 (75A:25W)

Practical uses: The essential oil of tea tree is the strongest antiseptic produced by plants, demonstrating broad-spectrum antimicrobial activity against bacteria, yeast, and viruses.

External: The high-alcohol tincture captures a sufficient quantity of the essential oil to make it a useful disinfectant for wounds and a valuable external application against acne, ringworm, athlete's foot, bacterial infections, candida, skin disease, canker sores, dental caries, bites, and stings. To repel head lice, apply to hair.

Douche: Dilute 2 droppersful (60 drops) of the tincture in 2 cups (480 ml) of warm water to make a useful vaginal douche against vaginitis caused by bacteria or yeast.

Poultice: The Australian aborigines used the crushed leaves as an antiseptic and healing poultice, and also inhaled the crushed leaves as a decongestant. These uses are still quite applicable, but require large quantities of the valuable leaves, which can probably only be efficiently produced by gardeners in the South.

Contraindications: The pure essential oil of tea tree contains cineole—a recognized skin irritant. The essential oil should always be diluted in a neutral base such as olive oil before applying to the skin. Tinctures of the leaves do not contain sufficient cineole to pose any hazard for external application. Internal use of tea tree is not recommended, as it can cause gastrointestinal irritation. Large quantities of the essential oil taken internally can potentially damage the kidneys.

276

Thistle, Blessed (*Cnicus benedictus*)
Family: Aster (*Asteraceae*)

Parts used: Whole aerial parts, including leaf, stem, and immature flowers, harvested in early flowering stage and used fresh or dried. In a single growing season, 2 cuttings can usually be made.

Tincture of fresh herb: 1:2 (75A:25W)

Tincture of dry herb (preferred): 1:5 (50A:50W)

Water extracts: Cold infusion of dry herb. Basic tea of fresh or dried herb.

Practical uses: The cold tea of blessed thistle is a valuable bitter tonic, improving appetite and helping with the assimilation of fats. The warm tea will produce a sweat that is of use in bringing down fevers. The herb is also a strong galactagogue, used for improving milk production and letdown reflex during nursing. Blessed thistle combines well with anise or fennel.

Dosage: According to basic recommendations found under "Dosage of tinctures," pages 49–52 and "Dosage of teas and decoctions," pages 70–71. As a bitter tonic, best taken just prior to meals.

Contraindications: Not to be used during pregnancy or in the presence of overt liver disease. High dosage may cause stomach upset or vomiting. Rare allergic reactions have been recorded.

Thistle, Milk (*Silybum marianum*)
Family: Aster (*Asteraceae*)

Parts used: Seed harvested when mature and dried. Sprouts, or fresh young leaves divested of the spines.

Tincture of dried seed: 1:3 (100A)
Grind the seeds before adding the alcohol. The active constituents (flavonolignans) reside mainly in the inner seed coat.

Water extracts: Not very useful, unless the seed is ground and the dregs consumed.

Direct consumption (preferred): The seeds are ground in an electric coffee mill or grain-grinding mill and taken plain, mixed into yogurt, or sprinkled on cereal. They are a bit too hard to be chewed up whole by any save those boasting of a bovine heritage. The whole seeds are naturally protected against rancidity, but the seed flour can easily go rancid—therefore, the seeds need to be stored whole and ground only as needed. The dosage is 1 tablespoonful (~8 g) twice daily, which is equivalent to a daily intake of 400 mg of pure silymarin (but better, due to the superiority of the whole herb that represents the entire array of constituents). The sprouted seeds and young, fresh leaves (divested of spines) provide a gentle stimulant to the liver and bile and are quite good in salads. However, cutting around the margins of fresh milk thistle leaves with scissors is a bit of a chore. Dandelion leaves are therapeutically interchangeable and much friendlier.

Practical uses: Milk thistle seed protects the liver from toxic substances and stimulates the regeneration of liver tissue in recuperation from hepatitis and alcoholism. The herb is especially indicated for people living in or working around environmental toxicity, including industrial pollution, radiation, hydrocarbon fumes, and bad water.

Dosage: According to basic recommendations found under "Dosage of tinctures," pages 49–52 and "Dosage of teas and decoctions," pages 70–71.

Contraindications: None known. Safe for general use. A mild laxative effect may be noticed.

278

Thyme (*Thymus vulgaris*)
Family: Mint (*Lamiaceae*)

Part used: Leaves harvested just prior to the plants' flowering, in the afternoon of a warm day, removed from the stems, and used fresh or dried.

Tincture of fresh herb: 1:2 (100A)

Tincture of dried herb: 1:5 (75A:25W)

Acetum of dried herb: 1:7 (100ACV); see page 55.

Water extract: Basic tea of fresh or dried leaves.

Practical uses: Thyme is a good astringent and an active antiseptic, most useful for treating upper respiratory infection— either viral or bacterial. The herb allays cough and bronchitis.

Dosage: According to basic recommendations found under "Dosage of tinctures," pages 49–52, and "Dosage of teas and decoctions," pages 70–71. Also see "Dosage of dry herb aceta," pages 55–56.

Food use: As a culinary spice, the fresh or dried leaf is added to food near the end of preparation, due to the presence of volatile oils. Thyme is very tasty on vegetarian, cheese, and meat dishes and is considered especially appropriate for seasoning eggs. The British are fond of using it on mutton.

Contraindications: The tea and tincture are safe for general use. Do not take the pure essential oil of thyme internally. Avoid direct contact with pure, undiluted essential oil of thyme, especially on sensitive skin, mucous membranes, and in eyes.

Other species: There are nearly 400 species in the *Thymus* genus, most of which exhibit culinary and medicinal attributes. These include: creeping thyme *(T. serphyllum),* mastic thyme (*T. mastichina*), and other wild-derived species. *T. vulgaris* is the official species, represented by several tasty cultivars, including: English broadleaf, French, and German winter thyme.

Tulsi (Holy Basil, Tulasi)
(*Ocimum sanctum* syn. *O. tenuiflorum*)
Family: Mint (*Lamiaceae*)

Parts used: The leaf and flowering tops, without the woody stem, harvested during the early flowering stage and used fresh or dried. The dried seeds. The dried root.

Tincture of fresh leaf and flower: 1:2 (75A:25W)

Tincture of dried leaf and flower: 1:5 (50A:50W)

Water extracts: Tea of the dried leaves and flowers or decoction of the dried root pieces or powdered roots.

Succus or syrup of fresh leaves and flowers: Use basic formulas found in "Chapter 9, Herbal Succi and Syrups." The succus has a blood-cleansing influence, and may be taken internally and used externally at the same time for treating ringworm, skin lesions, and eruptions. The succus is also used internally for treating colic, earache, fever, vomiting, intestinal worms, poisons, and shock. The fresh juice (without alcohol as a preservative) is similarly employed. The syrup is useful in treating upper respiratory infections (dispelling catarrh and allaying cough) and assists in rehabilitation of energy reserves after debilitating illness.

Traditional uses: According to ancient folklore, the tulsi (tulasi) plant is a manifestation of the Divine Mother on Earth, here for the benefit of all creation. The fragrant leaves and flowers, in the form of tincture, tea, or decoction, serve to sharpen the mind and are also considered to be stomachic and expectorant; used in treating indigestion, diarrhea, coughs, bronchitis, and skin diseases. These preparations are considered to be prophylactic against epidemics, such as cholera, influenza, and malaria. The seeds, taken mixed in water, juice, or cow's milk, are antioxidant, nourishing, mucilaginous, and demulcent—used in treating low energy, ulcers, vomiting, and diarrhea. The powder of the dried root, taken in milk, ghee, or as a decoction, is recommended to treat malarial fever and also to increase sexual stamina—preventing premature ejaculation. This powder may be made into a paste with water and used as an analgesic application to insect bites and stings.

Contemporary uses: Tulsi is a gentle and easy-to-grow adaptogen, meaning that the tea or tincture helps reduce the deleterious effects of stress, both physical and psychological. The plant enhances physical and mental endurance by optimizing assimilation of oxygen and nutrients to the bloodstream. Strong antioxidant activity slows the aging process and helps prevent and treat cancer, heart disease, arthritis, diabetes, and dementia. The herb normalizes blood pressure, blood sugar, and reduces LDL (so-called "bad") cholesterol. A morning cup of tulsi tea is an excellent wellness drink to help quit drinking coffee and reduce anxiety. The herb is also used during sickness to overcome cough, cold, flu, and fever. Tulsi assists digestion, tastes good and provides gentle stimulation to body, mind, and spirit.

Dosage: According to basic recommendations found under "Dosage of tinctures," pages 49–52 and "Dosage of teas and decoctions," pages 70–71. The dosage of the seed is 1 to 2 grams daily, and the dosage of the powdered root is 3 to 5 grams daily.

Contraindications: None known. Safe for general use.

Other species: Basils fall into two categories: the culinary basils (e.g. *Ocimum basilicum,* the essence of pesto), and the tea basils, which are better known for their medicinal attributes. Holy basil (*O. sanctum* syn. *O. tenuiflorum*) is the best of all tea basils. All types contain eugenol (which makes them smell like cloves) and rosmarinic acid (which is indicative of the anti-anxiety aspects of the herb). Amrita tulsi is a colorful, small-leaved type that is perennial in southern India and overwinters readily in a greenhouse in the temperate north. This is the most potent tulsi we have tested. Rama tulsi is nearly as potent, with leaves of green. Krishna tulsi, with its showy dark red or purple foliage, makes strong tea and is preferred by many. Kapoor tulsi is fruitily fragrant and easy to grow as a summer annual, making this gentle medicine one of the best choices for growers in the temperate north. Vana tulsi (*O. gratissimum*) is a tall, perennial bush basil with soft, tomentose leaves that covers a wide range as a roadside shrub in India and East Africa. Analysis of this highly productive species shows presence of eugenol as well as rosmarinic acid. This helps validate the traditional use of vana tulsi in tulsi tea blend.

𝒰

Unicorn, False (Helonias Root) (*Chamaelirium luteum*)
Family: Lily (*Liliaceae*)

Part used: Rhizome (the root) dug during dormancy and used fresh or dried. Since the herb is evergreen, "dormancy" refers to the resting period between fall and very early spring. The plant may be identified by the characteristic rosette of spatulate leaves. Winter harvest also gives the plant one last chance to make seeds. If seeds are present at harvest, rake away the garden mulch, crush up the seed heads, plant the seeds, and replace the mulch on top of the planting.

Fresh root: 1:2 (75A:25W) Given the at-risk status (fast disappearing from the wilds) of false unicorn, it is recommended to make the tincture from the fresh root, which stretches the medicine.

Dried root: 1:5 (50A:50W)

Water extracts: Basic tea or decoction of the fresh or dried root.

Practical uses: False unicorn is a good tonic for women. The herb regulates the menstrual cycle, improves the tone of the uterus and bladder, protects against uterine prolapse, and may improve fertility and act as an aphrodisiac for both men and women.

Dosage: According to basic recommendations found under "Dosage of tinctures," pages 49–52 and "Dosage of teas and decoctions," pages 70–71. Do not exceed recommended dosage.

Contraindications: Although a small amount of the extract in combination with other herbs is probably safe during pregnancy, false unicorn is a uterine stimulant and should not be taken alone—even at moderate dosage—during pregnancy.

Adulteration: False unicorn (*Chamaelirium luteum*) is not to be confused with true unicorn (*Aletris farinosa*). Adding to this confusion is the fact that true unicorn is also sometimes called false unicorn. These plants are botanically dissimilar, but are used to treat the same set of symptoms and have been substituted for each other in herbal trade.

Uva-Ursi (Bearberry, Kinnikinnick)
(*Arctostaphylus uva-ursi*)
Family: Heath (*Ericaceae*)

Parts used: The leaves, harvested any time by snipping the runner from the crown of the plant and gently stripping off the leaves. Rough handling causes them to darken. Lay out on screens in the shade, turning occasionally to encourage even dehydration. Store the dried leaves in whole form, in a sealed container, kept cool and out of the light. Just prior to extraction, crush the leaves or grind to a coarse powder.

Tincture of dried herb: 1:5 (60A:30W:10GLY) Combine (50:50) with marshmallow tincture for best results.

Water extracts: Cold infusion of dried herb. Containing up to 40% of tannins, uva-ursi preparations can cause gastric upset. For this reason, the cold infusion, which effectively extracts the glycosidal arbutin while leaving much of the hot water soluble tannin in the herb, is the preferred approach. Therapeutically, uva-ursi combines very well with marshmallow, which is also best extracted by means of the cold infusion. Make the infusions separately and then combine (50:50) before use.

Practical uses: Uva-ursi is a diuretic and urinary tract antiseptic used for treating urinary tract infections (UTI). Symptoms include constant urge to pee, frequent urination, itching or burning sensations, or pain in the genitourinary tract. Taking the tea or tincture of uva-ursi flushes the urinary tract, tonifies the urinary organs, and kills pain. The herb also delivers the precursor compound arbutin, which is absorbed through the gut into the bloodstream, then is filtered out again by the kidneys. From there the arbutin moves to the bladder, where it breaks down into hydroquinone, a powerful antibacterial agent that kills *Escherichia coli*, the most frequent pathogen involved in UTI.

The bladder environment must be alkaline in order for this process to occur. Since the presence of bacteria in the urinary tract promotes alkalinity, and uva-ursi itself is alkalinizing to the bladder, then nothing more need be done to assure alkalinity. However, foods and drinks that acidify the urine should be

283

avoided. These include refined sugar, processed carbohydrates, animal protein, tomatoes, alcoholic beverages, and coffee. Foods and drinks that hydrate the system and alkalinize the urine will promote the antibacterial effects of uva-ursi. These include pure water, leafy greens, fruits, whole grains, nuts, pumpkin seeds, and dairy products (especially yogurt and other probiotics). This diet will also help alleviate post-infection discomfort and limit recurrence.

Dosage: Of the tincture, 20 to 50 drops up to 5 times per day, best before meals. Of the cold infusion, 1 cup up to 5 times a day, best before meals. Combine with marshmallow for maximum comfort. This is the dosage for treatment of acute UTI, and should be maintained only for as long as necessary to banish the infection.

Contraindications: Taking uva-ursi may cause a darkening of the urine, which can be alarming, but is actually harmless. The high tannin content may cause gastric distress in predisposed individuals. If symptoms such as high fever, chills, nausea, or vomiting accompanied by back pain occur, this is a sign of a kidney infection, which is potentially life-threatening. Kidney infections are not treated by uva-ursi—seek professional help.

Other species: There are over a hundred species and subspecies in the *Arctostaphylos* genus, represented mainly by the smooth-stemmed dryland shrubs known as manzanita. These are closely allied to uva-ursi. Like our herb, their leaves contain substantial amounts of arbutin and tannin. Therefore, in a pinch, manzanita may be substituted for uva-ursi. American cranberry (*Vaccinium macrocarpon*) is another herb in the heath family that contains arbutin in its leaves. However, it is the fruit juice of the cranberry that holds a reputation for treating UTI. The procyanidins in cranberries acidify the urine and inhibit bacterial adhesion to the walls of the urinary tract, making bacteria easier to expel. Since the acid environment prohibits hydroquinone synthesis, cranberry juice is not a good choice for combining with uva-ursi therapy. However, drinking cranberry juice does help alleviate post-infection discomfort, and may prevent recurrence of UTI.

V

Valerian (*Valeriana officinalis*)
Family: Valerian (*Valerianaceae*)

Parts used: Root and rhizome (the root) harvested from fall to early spring and used fresh or dried.

Tincture of fresh herb (preferred): 1:2 (100A)

Tincture of recently dried herb: 1:5 (75A:25W)

Glycerite of fresh herb: 1:2 (100Gly)

Water extracts: Tea or decoction of fresh or recently dried roots.

Practical uses: Valerian is a sedative and also helps induce sleep. The herb can reduce stress, nervousness, and irritability.

Dosage: According to basic recommendations found under "Dosage of tinctures," pages 49–52 and "Dosage of teas and decoctions," pages 70–71. See also "Dosage of glycerites," page 63.

Contraindications: Safe for occasional use. Valerian is not a reliable sedative for all individuals, as some people actually experience nervous excitation from using this herb. Headaches are an occasional side effect. Overdose can cause drowsiness the following day. Some people experience bad dreams or nightmares from using valerian, others not; combination with passionflower tends to prevent bad dreams.

Other species: There are over 200 species in the *Valeriana* genus found worldwide. These include cape valerian (*V. capensis*) of South Africa, Indian valerian (*V. jatamansii)* of the Himalayas, and several species indigenous to North America, including the fairly well-known and potent Sitka valerian (*V. sitchensis*). Wild stands of valerian are sensitive to harvest. Domestication and cultivation of all useful species is a good priority. Meanwhile, *V. officinalis* can be readily cultivated. By the way, valerian is not to be confused with so-called "American valerian," the several kinds of lady's slipper orchid (*Cypripedium* spp.).

Vervain, Blue (*Verbena officinalis, V. hastata*)
Family: Vervain (*Verbenaceae*)

Parts used: Leaves and buds, without the stem, used fresh or dried.

Tincture of fresh herb: 1:2 (75A:25W)

Tincture of dried herb (preferred): 1:5 (50A:50W)

Water extract: Basic tea of dried herb.

Practical uses: Blue vervain is intensely bitter and, as such, will improve sluggish digestion. The herb is sedative to the nerves and is sometimes effective against headache. The tea or tincture is also taken hot to sweat out a fever, for treating colds and flu, and makes an effective galactagogue for increasing milk production in lactating mothers.

Dosage: According to basic recommendations found under "Dosage of tinctures," pages 49–52 and "Dosage of teas and decoctions," pages 70–71. As a bitter, best taken 15 to 20 minutes before meals.

Poultice: The poultice of the mashed, fresh plant can be applied to ease muscle soreness or the pain of rheumatism and to speed healing of wounds, burns, and lesions.

External: The strong tea is useful for making a sitz bath for treating hemorrhoids.

Contraindications: Not to be used during pregnancy or in the presence of overt liver disease.

Other species: There are about 200 species in the *Verbena* genus occurring worldwide, many of which are considered to be valuable medicinal plants, with uses ranging from treating urinary gravel to treating intestinal worms. A few of the species indigenous to North America are used interchangeably with the European *V. officinalis*, including *V. hastata*, *V. macdougalii*, *V. stricta*, and *V. bracteata*. Horticultural varieties and many of the spreading ground cover type vervains are very pretty, but not useful as medicinals.

Violet (*Viola odorata, V. tricolor*)
Family: Violet (*Violaceae*)

Parts used: Aerial portions of the plant picked in early flowering stage, including stems, leaves, and flowers, used fresh or dried. Sweet violet (*Viola odorata*) is considered to be stronger medicine than heartsease violet (*V. tricolor*), which is quite gentle.

Tincture of fresh herb: 1:2 (75A:25W)

Tincture of dried herb: 1:5 (50A:50W)

Water extract: Tea of the fresh or dried leaves and flowers.

Succus of fresh herb: 1 part alcohol by volume:3 parts juice by volume (see "Chapter 9, Herbal Succi and Syrups").

Syrup: Combine 1 part by volume of a strong decoction of the fresh or dried herb:2 parts by volume of honey (see page 77).

Practical uses: The herb is cooling and healing, mild enough for treating upper respiratory infection and cough of children, yet is a sufficiently persistent alterative to effectively treat chronic disease of adults—including even oral cancers.

Dosage: According to basic recommendations found under "Dosage of tinctures," pages 49–52.

External: The tea or tincture may be applied directly to the skin as a compress or a wash. This assists in resolving skin disorders of children—including rashes, cradle cap, and hives. Alcoholic extracts are diluted at the rate of 1 dropperful (30 drops) per ½ cup (120 ml) of water before using on mucous membranes.

Poultice: Violet leaves are mashed or bruised and applied cold, or mixed with a little hot water and ground flaxseed, for a healing and drawing poultice.

Oil, salve, or cream: Make an infused herbal oil of the fresh or dried violet leaves and/or flowers, then proceed to make salve according to the procedure found in "Chapter 10, Basic Formulas for Herbal Oils, Salves, and Creams." These products are good for moisturizing, toning, and healing the skin.

Contraindications: None known. Safe for general use.

W

Wild Yam, American (*Dioscorea quaternata, D. villosa*)
Family: Yam (*Dioscoraceae*)

Parts used: Whole rhizome and roots (the root) dug in dormancy and thinly sliced while still fresh, then dried before extraction.

Tincture of the dried root: 1:5 (50A:50W)
Due to the hardness of the root, macerating time needs to be extended to 5 weeks with daily agitation.

Water extract: Basic decoction of the ground or finely chopped, dried root.

Practical uses: American wild yam is generally used for allaying pain, being a progesterone precursor and an antispasmodic for smooth muscles of stomach, colon, ovaries, and uterus. The indications for using wild yam are acute abdominal pain, pain caused by gallstones, flatulence, spasmodic hiccups, menstrual cramps, pain and nausea during pregnancy, or rheumatic pain arising from liver and intestinal malfunction.

Dosage: According to basic recommendations found under "Dosage of tinctures," pages 49–52 and "Dosage of teas and decoctions," pages 70–71.

Contraindications: Extracts of the dried root are safe for general use. The roots must always be dried before extraction. Ingestion of fresh roots may cause irritation of mucous membranes, nausea, and/or emesis. Overdose of the dried root may also cause emesis. Although wild yam itself in cream form has little or no physiological affect, taking the herb internally over time will promote progesterone. Most wild yam products on the market contain synthetic progesterone. Synthetic progesterone in cream form does indeed have an immediate hormonal influence.

Wilde Dagga (*Leonotis leonurus*)
Family: Mint (*Lamiaceae*)

Parts used: Roots, leaves, and flowers harvested in the early flowering phase and used fresh or dried.

Tincture of the dried leaves or dried leaves and flowers: 1:5 (75A:25W)

Water extracts: Tea or decoction of the dried leaves and flowers.

Practical uses: The herb is used internally for treating upper respiratory infection, fever, headache, and high blood pressure.

Dosage: According to basic recommendations found under "Dosage of tinctures," pages 49–52 and "Dosage of teas and decoctions," pages 70–71.

External: The tea, decoction, or dilute tincture can be used as a pain-relieving, anti-itch, and healing wash or compress for treating skin conditions, such as oily skin, acne, and eczema.

Poultice: The fresh leaves and roots are mashed or pounded to make a pain-relieving and anti-inflammatory poultice for treating venomous bites and insect stings.

Smoking: The dried leaves are smoked. The effect is mildly euphoric and antispasmodic.

Contraindications: Although the herb is considered safe for internal use and the poultice is completely harmless, habitual smoking can be injurious.

Other species: Cordao (*Leonotis nepetaefolia*) is very similar to wilde dagga in many respects, with identical inflorescences, but different shaped leaves. Cordao is an annual, while wilde dagga is perennial. Both of these are showy hummingbird attractors.

Willow (*Salix* spp.)
Family: Willow (*Salicaceae*)

Parts used: The bark, stripped from twig and branch in the spring, when the sap is up. Small branches may be cut from the tree without harm, or use the two-year-old or older whips that rise up from the stump of a tree that has been previously cut or burned. Depending on the age and toughness of the tree, the bark may be peeled with thumbnail or shaved off with a knife. For fresh use, the bark must be processed quickly, as it dries rapidly. To dry, pile the quills on a screen in a warm, dark, airy location and turn frequently until they are thoroughly dehydrated. Store in a sealed container, out of the light, and grind to a coarse powder just prior to extraction.

Tincture of fresh bark: 1:3 (40A:50W:10GLY) Snip the pieces into short lengths with scissors, then use the blender method, p. 22.

Tincture of dried bark: 1:5 (30A:60W:10GLY) Salicin is water soluble. The glycerin stabilizes the tannins, which increases the shelf-life of the extract.

Water extracts: Tea or decoction of the fresh or dried bark. Steep the tea for at least 10 minutes. Milk may be added to bind the tannins and reduce incidence of stomach upset.

Practical uses: Willow bark contains the bitter glucoside known as salicin. When ingested, this compound is converted, by means of digestive hydrolysis and enzyme activity, into the anti-inflammatory and pain-relieving compound salicylic acid. The main use of willow bark extracts is in pain relief, including treatment of headache, lower back pain, other body aches, menstrual cramps, influenza, and rheumatic pain. Willow bark also contains very high concentrations (up to 20%) of polyphenolic tannins and flavonoids, including catechins. These compounds contribute to the analgesic effects. Willow bark tea or the dilute tincture may be applied externally as an astringent wash that will deaden pain and speed healing of ulcerations and wounds. The powerfully astringent, free radical scavenging, and antioxidant properties of the herb make it a potential candidate for treatment of cancerous tumors.

Dosage: According to basic recommendations found under "Dosage of tinctures," pages 49–52 and "Dosage of teas and decoctions," pages 70–71. The tannins in willow bark delay absorption of salicylates, therefore the herbal extracts take longer to work than aspirin. Willow bark extract may take 45 minutes to deaden pain, with maximum efficacy at 2 hours. The analgesic effect lasts for up to 4 hours. The minimum effective dosage will depend on the strength of the willow bark being used and the sensitivity of the patient. See "Other species."

Contraindications: The high tannin content of willow extracts may cause stomach upset or nausea in predisposed individuals. Not to be used during pregnancy or nursing. Individuals with known hypersensitvity to aspirin may react similarly to willow. Avoid taking willow for any conditions or diseases wherein aspirin is contraindicated. If fever is present, or if the child is recuperating from chicken pox or other viral infections, do not give willow, due to increased risk of Reye's syndrome (potentially life-threatening swelling of liver and brain).

Other species: When you know willow, you know variation— there are 350 species in *Salix*. They all contain salicin, but the actual content of active constituent will vary between the different species, will vary within each species, and is dependent on season of harvest, age of the tree, harvest method, and the efficiency of post-harvest processing of the bark. Weeping willow (*S. babylonica*) contains 3 to 4% salicin. Weeping willow works! I have seen good results from a simple tea made of spring harvested bark. White willow (*Salix alba*) is more or less official, but is widely inconsistent in its salicin content (1.5 to 11%). The purple osier willow (*S. purpurea*) is among the strongest worldwide, a recommended species to grow and keep in the medicinal garden, with salicin content ranging from 4 to 8%. The American black willow (*S. nigra*) is also rich in salicin, and is successfully employed as an analgesic by rootsy herbalists in the US, who know how to give a dose, determine the efficacy, and proceed accordingly.

Witch Hazel (*Hamamelis vernalis, H. virginiana*)
Family: Witch Hazel (*Hamamelidaceae*)

Parts used: Leaves and young twigs or dried bark, fresh or dried.

Tincture of fresh herb: 1:2 (65A:25W:10Gly)

Tincture of dried herb: 1:5 (50A:40W:10Gly)

Water extracts: Basic tea or decoction of the fresh or dried herb.

Witch hazel extract is a clear distillate containing 14% alcohol, a common remedy that can be purchased at any drugstore. The distillate is made from the partially-dried twigs of the plant, and is used externally to cool and shrink inflamed tissues. Witch hazel extract also makes an excellent solvent for jewelweed tincture. See page 203.

Practical uses: Taken internally, witch hazel is an anti-inflammatory and hemostatic, usually used to help arrest bleeding of the stomach, lungs, or other internal organs. The astringent action makes it a valuable treatment for diarrhea and dysentery.

Dosage: According to basic recommendations found under "Dosage of tinctures," pages 49–52 and "Dosage of teas and decoctions," pages 70–71.

External use: For treating varicose veins and spider veins, freely rub the water extract or the full-strength tincture into the affected area. A sitz bath prepared from the strong decoction diluted in 1 or 2 gallons of tepid water will help heal the perineal area in the case of postpartum trauma or stitches; this is also useful for treating hemorrhoids (see pages 100–101). A compress of the tea or the tincture diluted at the rate of 2 droppersful (60 drops) in 1 cup (240 ml) of water can also be helpful for treating the same conditions.

Poultice: The bruised or mashed leaves are applied for the astringent, shrinking, and drawing effect on swellings, tumors, stings, or venomous bites.

Contraindications: Not for extended internal use, since the tannins present in witch hazel, especially the concentrated form found in the bark, can cause stomach upset and can stress the liver.

Wood Betony (*Stachys officinalis*)
Family: Mint (*Lamiaceae*)

Part used: Leaves, without the woody stems and without the nearly scentless flowers, used fresh or dried.

Tincture of fresh herb (preferred): 1:2 (75A:25W)

Tincture of dried herb: 1:5 (50A:50W)

Water extracts: Tea of fresh leaves, finely sliced or minced (preferred). Tea of dried leaves.

Practical uses: Wood betony is a nervine tonic and pain-reliever, good for treating nerve pain, toothache, and headache. The herb supports recuperation from chronic disease or addiction. Wood betony was once considered a panacea and, in my personal experience, this is not far from true. Traditional uses range from treating battle wounds to protecting against the plague.

Dosage: According to basic recommendations found under "Dosage of tinctures," pages 49–52 and "Dosage of teas and decoctions," pages 70–71.

Poultice: The fresh, bruised or mashed leaves make a healing and pain-relieving poultice for treating cuts, bruises, swellings, painful joints, splinters, or ulcerations.

Contraindications: None known. Safe for general use.

Other species: Much confusion surrounds the identification of herbs known as "betony." Wood betony must not be confused with members of the *Pedicularis* genus, which are also commonly known as "betony." The correct Latin name for wood betony is *Stachys officinalis*, a synonym of *Betonica officinalis* and *Stachys betonica*. This herb is also known as "common betony." Hedge nettle (*Stachys rigida*) is a potent-smelling herb of moist forestlands, that has a wide distribution in the mountains of the Pacific Northwest. This plant is used by locals as an analgesic and astringent, especially for treating headache and sore throat. My children once dubbed it "stink mint." Other species in the *Stachys* genus are also healers, including wooly lamb's ears (*S. byzantina*), as well as various woundworts: *S. germanica*, *S. palustris*, *S. recta*, and *S. sylvatica*.

293

Wormwood (*Artemisia absinthium*)
Family: Aster (*Asteraceae*)

Parts used: Leaves and flowers harvested in early flowering stage, without the stems, used dried or (sparingly) fresh.

Tincture of dried herb: 1:5 (50A:50W)

Water extracts: Cold infusion of dried herb. Basic tea of dried herb. Weak tea of fresh herb.

Direct consumption: Chew a fresh leaf.

Practical uses: Wormwood is the bitterest of all herbs. The tea or tincture forms a digestive bitter which, when taken before meals, markedly improves appetite and digestion. The herb tonifies both the stomach and the gallbladder. Wormwood is also a general antiparasitic used for treating a wide variety of parasites, including pinworms.

Dosage: According to basic recommendations found under "Dosage of tinctures," pages 49–52 and "Dosage of teas and decoctions," pages 70–71. This herb is not for long-term use and is somewhat self-limiting, since after one or several weeks, the bitter taste becomes (shudder) repugnant. At this milepost, the bitters have generally done their work, and it is time to discontinue the therapy.

Contraindications: Not to be used during pregnancy. The fresh herb, and products made from it, can be nauseating, which is why the dried herb is preferred. Wormwood contains thujone, which is a convulsant poison if taken in large doses. This is normally not a concern with teas and tinctures, but is a definite reason to avoid internal use of the distilled essential oil. Avoid direct contact with pure, undiluted essential oil of wormwood, especially on sensitive skin, mucous membranes, and in eyes.

Processing cautions: When grinding or otherwise handling large quantities of the dried herb, a filter mask should be worn.

Other species: The *Artemisia* genus is represented by about 200 species, many of which are good digestive bitters. These include Roman wormwood (*A. ponticus*), mugwort (*A. vulgaris*), and southernwood (*A. abrotanum*). See "*Artemisia annua*."

$\mathcal{Y}$

Yarrow (*Achillea millefolium*)
Family: Aster (*Asteraceae*)

Parts used: The flowers or the whole aerial parts harvested in the flowering stage and used fresh or dried.

Fresh herb: 1:2 (100A)

Dried herb: 1:5 (75A:25W)

Water extracts: Basic tea of fresh or dried herb.

Practical uses: Yarrow is a classic hemostatic and antiseptic used for treating bleeding, whether from internal causes or from deep wounds. It is also a bitter tonic and an antispasmodic, and will improve digestion if taken prior to the meal. Hot yarrow tea is also taken for treating colds and sweating out fever. The flowers are sometimes used in the manufacture of wine and beer.

Dosage: According to basic recommendations found under "Dosage of tinctures," pages 49–52 and "Dosage of teas and decoctions," pages 70–71.

External use: The full-strength tea or the tincture diluted at the rate of 1 dropperful (30 drops) in ½ cup (120 ml) of cold water can be used as an antiseptic compress or wash to bathe wounds, also serving to allay bleeding. A sitz bath prepared from the strong tea diluted in 1 or 2 gallons of tepid water can help reduce menstrual cramps.

Poultice: The bruised or mashed leaves make an excellent first aid poultice for treating traumatic injuries—especially deep cuts. Hikers and rock climbers would do well to know about this herb.

Oil, salve, or cream: Make an infused herbal oil of the bruised, fresh herb, then proceed to make salve or cream according to the procedure found in "Chapter 10, Basic Formulas for Herbal Oils, Salves, and Creams." The oil is useful for treating wounds and the cream is useful for tonifying the skin.

Contraindications: Not to be used during pregnancy. If use of yarrow causes skin inflammation or dermatitis, discontinue use. Avoid direct contact with pure, undiluted essential oil of yarrow, especially on sensitive skin, mucous membranes, and in eyes.

Cultivars: There are several different horticultural varieties of yarrow, including "rosea," "cerise queen," etc. Medicinally, these are far inferior to the wild, white-flowered yarrow. In order to grow yarrow that yields a potent medicine, plant the official variety in poor soil and water sparingly. Giving yarrow stressful growing conditions increases the essential oil content of the flowers.

Yellow Dock (Curly Dock) (*Rumex crispus*) Family: Buckwheat (*Polygonaceae*)

Parts used: Root dug during dormancy and dried. Fresh leaves for poulticing.

Tincture of dried root: 1:5 (50A:40W:10Gly)

Water extract: Decoction of the dried root.

Syrup: Combine 1 part by volume of a strong decoction of the dried roots:2 parts by volume of honey. Follow procedure found in "Chapter 9, Herbal Succi and Syrups."

Practical uses: The root is mildly laxative, useful in treating constipation and iron deficiency. Women use it during the menstrual period. The root also has a blood-cleansing effect, often combined with dandelion, chickweed, cleavers, and burdock to make a spring tonic. This helps dispel toxins from the system and improves oily skin and acne.

Dosage: According to basic recommendations found under "Dosage of tinctures," pages 49–52 and "Dosage of teas and decoctions," pages 70–71.

External: The full-strength decoction of yellow dock or the tincture diluted at the rate of 2 droppersful (60 drops) in 1 cup (240 ml) of cold water make a strong astringent that is used as a gargle for sore throat, improving the tone of boggy tissues and relieving pain. This can also be used externally as a wash or compress for reducing skin inflammation caused by insect bites or allergies.

Poultice: The fresh leaves are bruised or mashed and applied to swellings, oily skin, or cuts and scrapes, for the cleansing, astringent, and pain-relieving effects.

Contraindications: The herb is rich in tannins, sometimes measuring as high as 20%. Individuals with a history of kidney stones should probably not take it internally, or at least combine the decoction or dilute tincture with milk to bind the tannins before use. Overdose causes gastric irritation and diarrhea.

Other species: There is variation in the appearance of yellow dock (*Rumex crispus*) depending on locality. Some plants may have a flatter, lance-shaped leaf, while others will bear leaves with curly margins. These variations do not affect the medicinality of the plant. Yellow dock is identified by the presence of winged, heart-shaped seeds and a branching taproot that is yellow inside. One other species of note, which has much the same medicinal application as yellow dock, is the native southwestern plant known as canaigre (*R. hymenosepalus*). Dock is medicinally and botanically distinct from sorrel (*R. scutatus, R. acetosella*). These have sour-tasting leaves due to the presence of oxalic acid.

Yerba Mansa (*Anemopsis californica*)
Family: Lizard's Tail (*Saururaceae*)

Parts used: Rhizome (the root) dug any time and used fresh or dried. The leaves harvested at maturity and used fresh or dried.

Tincture of fresh root: 1:2 (90A:10Gly)

Tincture of dried root: 1:5 (75A:15W:10Gly)

Water extract: Basic tea or decoction of the fresh or dried root.

Direct consumption: Chew a bit of the fresh or dried root.

Practical uses: Yerba mansa is a good treatment for upper respiratory infection. It stimulates the immune response, fights infection, and helps to thin and dispel thick catarrh from the lungs, sinuses, and bronchi. The herb is a useful astringent for treating diarrhea and gastroenteritis.

Dosage: According to basic recommendations found under "Dosage of tinctures," pages 49–52 and "Dosage of teas and decoctions," pages 70–71.

External: The tincture diluted at the rate of 2 droppersful (60 drops) in 1 cup (240 ml) of warm water or the full-strength decoction make a disinfectant, astringent, and anti-inflammatory wash or compress for treating wounds. This dilute tincture also makes an effective gargle. A sitz bath prepared from the strong decoction diluted in 1 or 2 gallons of tepid water can help resolve vaginal or urinary infections.

Oil, salve, or cream: Make an infused herbal oil of the fresh or dried leaves, then make salve or cream according to the procedure found in "Chapter 10, Basic Formulas for Herbal Oils, Salves, and Creams." This is a useful disinfectant and healer for wounds, burns, and skin ulcerations.

Contraindications: None known. Safe for general use.

Glossary

The definitions given in this glossary are applicable within the context of this book and are of general utility in the understanding of herbalism and herbal pharmacy.

abortifacient: an agent that can cause accidental abortion of a fetus.

absorption: dermal absorption occurs when medicinal substances enter the body tissues and blood stream through the skin.

absolute alcohol: the pure alcohol content of any alcoholic beverage, menstruum, or tincture.

aceta: tinctures made with 100% vinegar as the menstruum.

acetic acid: a pungent, colorless liquid acid that is the chief acid agent in vinegar; molecular formula $C_2H_4O_2$.

acetous tincture: an alcoholic tincture, acidified by the addition of vinegar or acetic acid to the menstruum.

acetum: (*plural* aceta) a tincture made with 100% vinegar as the menstruum.

acidification: adding an acid substance to the menstruum in order to assist in extraction of alkaloids.

active constituent: a molecule or compound present in an herb that contributes to the medicinal effect (e.g. sanguinarine in bloodroot).

activity: the medicinal effect residing in an herb.

acute: short-lived but severe symptoms—the opposite of chronic.

ACV: abbreviation for apple cider vinegar.

adaptogenic: an herb that assists in adapting one to stress, whether emotional, physical, or environmental. The hallmark of adaptogens is that they have a *normalizing* influence on physiological processes.

adrenergic stimulant: an herb that stimulates the autonomic nerve endings by activating and transmitting adrenaline.

adulterant: In herbal trade, there is a universal expectation that the true identity of an herb is accurately represented by the claimed identity or labeling of that herb. If the package or shipment contains misidentified herbs, whether due to error in identification or purposeful substitution, the herbs are said to be adulterated. The misidentified herbs are an adulterant.

aerial: the aboveground portion of a plant, usually consisting of stems and leaves, often with buds, flowers, and/or seeds attached.

affect: to produce an influence upon or alteration in the body.

alcohol:water ratio: a volume:volume ratio describing the relative percentages of grain alcohol and distilled water used in the mixing of menstruum for herbal tincturing.

alkaloid: a class of biologically active, alkaline compounds that contain nitrogen in the molecule. Purified plant alkaloids are usually crystalline and white, with the notable exceptions of berberine (yellow) and sanguinarine (red).

alkaloidal herbs: herbs that contain one or more alkaloid(s) as the main active constituent.

alkaloidal salts: When an acid menstruum is poured over certain alkaloidal herbs, a reaction occurs wherein the alkaloids are turned into alkaloidal salts, which then become available to the tincture.

alkylamide: a type of active constituent found in echinacea that is responsible for the familiar oral "buzzing" sensation.

allopathic: relating to the current system of nonherbal medical practice.

alpha-linolenic: an omega-3 fatty acid as found in evening primrose, flaxseed, purslane, soy products, and dark green vegetables.

alterative: an herb or therapy that stimulates a material change in the underlying causes of chronic or acute disease symptoms, often by influencing glandular activity, thereby re-establishing healthy body function. Alteratives sometimes precipitate a healing crisis wherein chronic conditions become acute and are then banished.

analgesic: relieving pain. A remedy for pain.

antagonist: an herb that opposes the activity of another herb, a drug or an aspect of body chemistry, such as a hormone; i.e. "Bugleweed is a thyroxin antagonist."

anthraquinone laxative: an herbal laxative depending on plant glycosides (e.g. emodin, rhein) to produce cathartic activity. Absorption of the herb occurs only after the constituents are hydrolyzed in the small intestine, resulting in a delayed action.

anticancer: opposing the onset, development, or spread of malignant cells or tumors.

anthelmintic: destructive to intestinal worms.

antidepressant: an herb that lifts the spirits; elevates the mood; shifts the mind toward positive thoughts.

antiflatulent: improving digestion; lessening expulsion of gas.

antifungal: an herb (e.g. tea tree) that kills or resists the spread of fungal infections (e.g. ringworm, athlete's foot).

anti-inflammatory: an herb that reduces swelling and inflammation, either internal (e.g. wild yam) or external (e.g. arnica).

antimicrobial: an herb that kills or resists the spread of microbial organisms (germs).

antimitotic: an herb that arrests the process of cell division known as mitosis. This is significant therapy in cancer, where there is runaway cell division.

antioxidant: an herb that acts to protect the body cells against damage from free radicals; a cell protectant.

antiparasitic: an herb that kills or inhibits the spread of parasites.

antiseptic: an herb that prevents decay and putrefaction and kills or resists the spread of malevolent germs.

antispasmodic: an herb that relaxes muscle spasms.

antiviral: an herb that kills or inhibits the spread of viral organisms.

anxiolytic: anti-anxiety; calming to the nerves.

aphrodisiac: an herb that increases sexual desire and improves sexual performance.

aromatic: an herb having a strong fragrance, usually due to the presence of essential oils.

arrhythmia: any variation of rhythm in the beating of the heart (e.g. extrasystole, fibrillation, tachycardia).

arteriosclerosis: thickening and hardening of the arterial walls.

arthritis: inflammation of the joints characterized by pain, heat, redness, swelling, and reduced functionality.

assure: to make sure or certain.

astringent: causing contraction of tissues; lessening discharge.

atonic: without tone; tissues or organs lacking normal tension and elasticity, resulting in reduced functionality.

attention deficit disorder (ADD or ADHD): inattention, impulsiveness, and/or hyperactivity that affects learning and development.

autoimmune: an immune response of an organism that is antagonistic to any of its own tissues.

berberine: a bitter, yellow, isoquinoline alkaloid such as can be found in goldenseal (*Hydrastis canadensis*).

beta-asarone: a molecule found in calamus (*Acorus calamus*), which can be carcinogenic if taken in excess.

beta-sitosterol: a type of plant steroid (phytosterol) that has an inflammation-inhibiting effect. Beta-sitosterol is very concentrated in small-flowered-willow-herb.

binomial: in taxonomy, the system of naming plants wherein the first name identifies the genus to which the plant belongs and the second identifies the exact species (e.g. *Calendula officinalis*).

bitters: an unsweetened elixir containing aromatic and bitter herbs, which aids in digestion.

bolus: a rounded mass of medicinal material.

botanicals: a general term for medicines made from plants.

calyx: in botany, the outer enveloping leafy structure, often green but sometimes intensely colored, that clasps the base of the flower—the sepals.

canker sore: an ulceration inside the mouth or lips.

capping off: putting on the cap or lid.

capsaicin: an intensely pungent phenolic compound present in cayenne; molecular formula $C_{18}H_{27}NO_3$.

carbuncle: a subcutaneous inflammation giving rise to a polyheaded cyst.

cardioactive: having an influence on the heart muscle.

cardiotonic: having a tonifying influence on the heart muscle.

carminative: an herb that relieves indigestion and flatulence.

caries (dental): tooth decay.

chronic: a long-lived or recurring medical condition.

cineole: a constituent of many essential oils, including eucalyptus and tea tree oil; a recognized skin irritant.

cold-pressed fixed oil: an oil that is liquid at room temperature, obtained from vegetable sources by expressing under high pressure at relatively low temperature.

comminution: grinding.

compound tincture: 2 or more *single herb extracts* mixed together to make a compound designed to achieve a certain therapeutic goal; 2 or more herbs mixed together *prior to extraction* to make a compound.

concurrent: operating at the same time and acting in conjunction.

constituent: see "active constituent."

conjunctivitis: inflammation and infection of the mucous membranes around the eye—usually characterized by a purulent discharge.

contraindication: a condition under which the use of any particular herb or procedure is not advised.

Coumadin: a pharmaceutical drug containing the anticoagulant warfarin.

counterirritant: an agent that produces superficial irritation meant to relieve a condition (e.g. the external use of cayenne in order to increase peripheral circulation).

crude extract: an unfinished (unfiltered) tincture.

crystallization: the formation of solid crystals in a liquid.

curative: contributing to or used in the cure of disease.

decant: to pour or siphon clear liquid off the top of an extract without disturbing the bottom sediment.

decoction: a water extract of herbs made by first soaking, then simmering the ingredients.

deleterious: harmful, hurtful, noxious, or pernicious.

demulcent: a bland, soothing, often mucilaginous herb; the soothing *activity* of a demulcent herb.

dermatitis: inflammation of the skin, often accompanied by scaling and shedding of the outer skin layers.

diaphoretic: an herb that promotes sweating or perspiration; a sudorific.

diluted alcohol: a menstruum composed of 50% grain alcohol and 50% distilled water.

distillation: a process that involves driving vapor from liquids or solids, then condensing the vapor to form a purified liquid substance such as alcohol or essential oils.

distilled alcohol: alcohol obtained by the distillation of fermented liquor.

diuretic: an herb that increases the flow of urine.

dropperful: (*plural* droppersful) a unit of liquid measure consisting of ~30 drops from a standard glass dropper, which is equivalent to ~1 ml of liquid.

drying sample: a sample of fresh herb that is weighed in the fresh state, dried, and weighed again in order to determine the relative percentages of water and dry material in the herb.

duodenal: pertaining to the duodenum—the first proximal portion of the small intestine.

efficacy: the ability to produce a result; effectiveness.

emulsification: the dispersion of oil in a watery medium.

eczema: an inflammatory skin condition characterized by scaliness and exudation of lymph.

effect: a result produced by an agent or a cause.

emesis: vomiting

emetic: an herb that causes vomiting, usually only if used in high dosage or wrong form.

emmenagogue: an herb that stimulates the onset of menstruation.

emollient: an herb that softens, moistens, and protects the body tissues—especially the skin and the mucous membranes; the soothing *activity* of an emollient herb.

ensure: to make sure, certain, or safe.

error of parallax: When measuring, it is best to view the level of liquid in a graduated cylinder at eye level. Viewing from above causes error of parallax, resulting in inaccurate measurement.

escharotic: caustic; corrosive; causing sloughing of skin (e.g. bloodroot).

essential oils: aromatic terpenes; volatile oils found in many plants, freely soluble in alcohol and capable of being concentrated by distillation (e.g. lavender, rosemary, sage).

expectorant: an herb that assists in the expulsion of mucous from the lungs and upper respiratory tract.

express: to squeeze out under pressure.

extract: a liquid herbal extract, such as a tincture, tea, or decoction. Also the act of drawing out the active constituents from an herb by means of soaking in a liquid menstruum.

extractive: any agent derived from the herb through extraction.

fibrolinic: blood-thinning activity. An herb that discourages blood platelet aggregation (e.g. garlic).

finished extract: the completed tincture, after filtering.

flavonoid: a class of plant constituents that tend to strengthen the vascular system; colored compounds found in many flowers and fruits (e.g. calendula flowers, black elderberry fruits).

flatulence: excessive formation of gasses in the intestine and expulsion of same. Carminatives relieve flatulence.

fomentation: a warm, moist medicinal compress, such as a cotton cloth soaked in a strong decoction and held to an injury.

formulary: a listing of established modes of standard procedures; a recipe book for making medicine from a wide array of substances.

free radicals: unstable reactive molecules that can cause cellular damage and are often linked to cancer.

galactagogue: an herb that increases the flow of milk (e.g. fennel).

gangrene: progressive mortification and death of tissue.

gastric: pertaining to the stomach.

gastroenteritis: inflammation of the stomach and intestines, usually accompanied by pain, nausea, and diarrhea.

gastrointestinal: pertaining to the stomach and intestines.

genitourinary: pertaining to the genital and urinary organs.

Gly: abbreviation for glycerin.

glycerin: a syrupy liquid obtained from oils and fats that is used as a solvent, preservative, and stabilizer in tincture making.

glycerite: a liquid herbal extract made using glycerin as both solvent and preservative.

glycoside: A class of biologically active compounds consisting of glucose (the glycone) linked to an active constituent (the aglycone).

goiter: enlargement of the thyroid gland.

gout: a painful constitutional disease of the joints (and especially the big toe), characterized by episodes of swelling, caused by inefficient excretion and subsequent crystallization of uric acid in the joints.

grain alcohol: 190 proof distilled alcohol made from grain. Grain alcohol has an absolute alcohol content of 95%.

graduated cylinder: a measuring device for liquids; a column marked on the side with volumetric graduations.

Grave's disease: a severe complication of hyperthyroidism; thyrotoxicosis.

grinding: the act of reducing the particle size of herbs with a mill or a blender.

griping: an intense spasm of the smooth muscles of the intestines.

gynecological: of or relating to women and especially the reproductive organs of women.

halophytic: salt-loving plant.

herb: a plant or plant part used in herbal therapy.

herb:menstruum ratio: compares the weight of the herb to the volume of the total liquid menstruum.

homeopathic: an ethereal system of medical practice that treats disease by the administration of minute remedial doses.

homeostasis: a state of relative equilibrium and cooperation between the various interdependent organs in a living body.

hybridize: to produce plant hybrids, either by way of human intervention or in nature. F-1 hybrids (meaning first filial generation) are intentional crosses of unlike parent plants. These hybrids demonstrate uniformity and hybrid vigor, but their seed does not breed true to type. Natural hybrids occur between different species of a given plant genus in nature, by open-pollination. Natural hybridization results in variation, stability, and disease resistance in the population. The seed of these plants produces offspring that demonstrate the same healthy array of variation as the parents.

hyperactive: excessively or pathogenically active.

hypersensitivity: excessively or abnormally sensitive.

hypoactive: insufficiently active; functionally deficient.

hypotensive: an herb that tends to lower blood pressure.

hypothyroidism: deficient activity of the thyroid gland.

immune-enhancing: an herb that stimulates the immune response, thereby increasing general resistance to disease.

infused oils: herbal oils created by steeping herbs in vegetable oil for a period of time.

infusion: tea created by steeping or soaking herbs in water.

isoquinoline alkaloids: a class of medicinally active alkaloids including berberine, hydrastine, sanguinarine, emetine, and certain opium alkaloids.

larynx: a muscular and cartilaginous structure lined with mucous membrane, located in the upper trachea in humans, housing the vocal chords.

latent: present, but not visible or currently active.

laxative: an herb that helps soften the stools, increases peristalsis, and thereby assists in moving the bowels.

legion: multitudinous.

lesion: any sore, wound, ulceration, or localized degeneration of tissue.

letdown reflex: relaxation of the mammary glands allowing milk to freely flow.

linoleic acid: an essential fatty acid found in certain foods and herbs (e.g. flaxseed).

local effect: bringing about changes to a localized area (e.g. the skin of the wrist or the mucous membranes of the throat).

low-dose botanicals: herbs that are extremely active and must therefore be used at low dosage (e.g. 5 drops of the tincture diluted in water taken 3 times a day) in order to regulate their activity and reduce the possibility of side effects.

MAOIs: mono-amine oxidase inhibitors block the enzymatic break-down of neurotransmitters (chemical substances that transmit nerve impulses). Widely used in production of antidepressant drugs.

marc: the press-cake left over after pressing herbal extracts.

macerate: to soak ground or sliced herbs in the fluid menstruum for a period of time, thereby softening them and making the active constituents available to the tincture.

meniscus: the curved upper surface of a liquid column (e.g. alcohol in a graduated cylinder) that is concave when the walls of the container are wetted by the liquid and convex when the walls of the column are dry.

menopause: the period of natural cessation of menstruation occurring usually between the ages of 45 and 50.

menses: monthly menstrual period.

menstrual: of or relating to menstruation.

menstruum: a liquid solvent that is used to extract active constituents from an herb.

midrib: the central vein of a leaf.

mortification: necrosis; gangrene; death of living tissue.

mucilage: a slimy substance produced by plants—generally cleansing and soothing to the mucous membranes; gums.

mucilaginous: full of mucilage (e.g. marshmallow root).

mucous membrane: a sensitive membrane rich in mucous glands that lines the body passages and cavities (e.g. the lining of the gastro-intestinal tract).

*Mycoplasma***:** very tiny gram-positive bacteria responsible for a plethora of health woes and often associated with lyme disease.

nervine: an herb that helps tonify the nerves, usually allaying nervous excitement.

nontoxic: an herb or substance that is safe to use as directed.

normalizing: bringing organs or physiological processes into balance.

open-pollinated: a natural strain of plants that is allowed to freely pollinate between the members of the population, creating a diverse and stable gene pool—not genetically modified.

overdose: excessive dosage resulting in an unwanted and sometimes dangerous physiological response.

overindulgence: partaking of an herb or food with unrestrained pleasure, resulting usually in an uncomfortable bodily response (e.g. indigestion).

overwinter: the ability for plants to survive through the winter.

oxidation: a chemical degradation of a substance caused by exposure to oxygen in storage.

oxygen-labile constituents: active constituents that are unstable in the presence of oxygen.

oxytocin: a pituitary hormone that stimulates uterine contractility.

PA: abbreviation of pyrrolizidine alkaloid.

palliative: an herb that alleviates symptoms, but does not provide a cure.

panacea: a cure-all.

pantropical: across the tropical regions of the earth.

parboil: to immerse briefly in boiling water.

parasite: an organism that lives on or in another organism, deriving benefit without giving compensation, often to the detriment of the host.

partus praeparator: a substance that readies the uterus for childbirth.

pathogen: a disease-causing organism.

pharmaceutical grade: pure; suitable for use in pharmacy.

physiological: characteristic of or pertaining to the normal functioning of living organisms.

physiomedical tradition: a system of herbal medicine developed in the mid- to late-19th century based on the belief that each individual carries an inherent "vital force," a kind of cellular intelligence capable of orchestrating physiological functions.

plant constituents: active constituents contained in plants.

plantar warts: deeply embedded warts in the sole of the foot.

platens: platforms.

PMS: abbreviation for premenstrual syndrome.

polyacetylene: a class of plant constituents demonstrating potential immune-enhancing effects.

polysaccharides: a class of carbohydrate plant constituents which tend to be immune-stimulating and nutritive.

poultice: vegetable material, whole or mashed, which is layered or spread on the skin.

postpartum: after the process of giving birth to offspring.

precipitate: in an extract, to cause solid particles to fall out of solution.

precipitation: in an extract, the process wherein solid particles (often active constituents, sometimes inert) fall out of solution.

premenstrual syndrome (PMS): symptoms (usually emotional) experienced just prior to the onset of the menstrual cycle.

preservative: a substance used to prohibit growth of bacteria in liquid extracts (e.g. alcohol or glycerin).

pressing: the act of expressing liquid from the macerating herb.

pressing cloth: a high-tensile cloth designed for holding the herbal slurry during expression.

principle constituent: main active constituent.

procyanidin: a flavonoid constituent, also known as a bioflavan, that has positive effects on the vascular system. High quantities of procyanidins may be found in blue, purple and red berries (e.g. bilberries, elderberries, and hawthorn berries).

prophylactic: guarding from or preventing disease.

prostatitis: chronic inflammation of the prostate gland in association with noncancerous proliferation of cells, often associated with symptoms such as painful urination, frequent urination, urinary infection, blood in the urine and/or incontinence. This condition is also termed benign prostatic hypertrophy (BPH), and is often a precursor to more serious conditions, including cancer of the prostate.

psoriasis: a skin disease characterized by scaly, red patches.

purging: causing the bowels to evacuate with force; catharsis.

pyrrolizidine alkaloids (PAs): a group of alkaloids found mainly in members of the *Asteraceae* and *Boraginaceae* families (e.g. gravel root, comfrey), which are potentially toxic to the liver.

raceme: a spike or stalk upon which numerous flowers are borne on individual stems.

reclassified: classified again; changed in its classification.

render stable: to be made stable.

resins: a diverse class of sticky, oily, generally bioactive plant constituents that are soluble in alcohol.

resolvent: breaking down or dissipating pathologic growth; arresting the inflammatory process.

return: efficiency of extraction expressed as a percent.

rheumatic joints: body joints (e.g. elbow, knee) affected by recurrent swelling and pain.

rheumatic pain: pain associated with rheumatism.

rheumatism: a constitutional disease marked by inflammation and dull pain in the muscles and joints.

ringworm: a fungus infection (often contracted from cats), characterized by intensely itchy, raised, red rings on the surface of the skin.

rosette: a cluster of leaves in crowded circles or spirals arising basally from a crown.

rubefacient: an externally applied agent that brings circulation to the surface of the skin.

saliva: an alkaline secretion of the mouth, composed of water, mucin, protein, salts, and enzymes.

salivary glands: a set of glands located in the mouth, responsible for producing saliva.

saponins: water-soluble, glycosidal plant constituents, many with positive biological effects (e.g. ginseng, chickweed), but some causing the plant to be very soapy and indigestible or poisonous (e.g. soapwort).

sedative: an herb that calms, moderates, or tranquilizes nervousness or excitement.

seed precipitation: to initiate the process wherein solid particles (often active constituents, sometimes inert constituents) fall out of solution.

septicemia: a condition of morbidity wherein pathogenic bacteria invade the blood stream; blood-poisoning.

serous membranes: the lining membrane of any of the greater body organs or lymphatic cavities, which protects the organs from harm, but can sometimes become painfully inflamed (e.g. pleurisy).

settling: the process where a crude liquid extract is allowed to sit in order to separate out solid particles

sialagogue: an herb that stimulates the secretion of saliva (e.g. spilanthes).

slow transport time: slow digestion; constipation.

slurry: a watery or alcoholic mixture of mashed or blended plants, the macerating extract of fresh plants.

solubility: in tincture making, the extent to which an herb or an active constituent is dissolved by a given liquid solvent (alcohol, water, or both) at a given temperature. "Resinous herbs have high solubility in alcohol, while their solubility in water is very low."

soluble protein: a (usually) inert agent that is dissolved from the herb and may later precipitate out of solution (e.g. pectin).

solvent: the liquid menstruum, which becomes "loaded" with extractives from the herbs in the process of maceration.

spider veins: capillary blood vessels on the surface of the skin.

spreens: edible spring greens; spring shoots.

stimulant: an herb that produces a temporary increase in the functional activity of an organism (e.g. mint or tea).

styptic: an herb that arrests hemorrhage, usually by dint of its astringency (e.g. witch hazel); a hemostatic.

subcutaneous: situated or occurring beneath the skin.

succus: (*plural succi*) Latin for juice; also a term given to a preparation containing plant juice mixed with only sufficient alcohol to preserve it.

succussion: vigorous shaking. "The macerating extract is subjected to daily succussion for a period of 3 weeks."

sudorific: an herb that causes sweating; a diaphoretic.

suppuration: formation of, conversion into, or discharge of pus.

swelling factor: the degree to which a dry herbal substance expands when a liquid menstruum is added to it.

tannins: a class of active phenolic or flavonoid compounds that demonstrate positive biological activity. Tannins are produced by the plant as a protective mechanism and generally act on the human physiology by shrinking swollen or injured tissues and allaying pain.

tanshinone: a lipophilic diterpene quinone molecule that is the main active constituent of the Chinese herb dan-shen.

taxonomy: the science of identification, description, naming, and classification of biological organisms.

taxonomist: one who studies the natural relationships of plants and animals and creates orderly (usually hierarchical) classifications of the same. "The machinations of taxonomists are endless."

telomeric effect: protecting the chromosomes from age-related deterioration, which helps promote longevity.

tensile: of or relating to tension. "The polypropylene pressing cloth demonstrated high tensile strength—until the dandelion exploded."

terpenes: a class of aromatic plant constituents—the primary active ingredient in essential oils and resins.

thiosulfinate: Raw garlic cloves and sun-macerated garlic oil, as well as the tincture of raw garlic, contain thiosulfinate compounds that exhibit marked antibacterial effect.

thrombophlebitis: inflammation of the blood vessels accompanied by obstructive (and potentially dangerously mobile) blood clots.

thyroxin: the iodine-containing hormone secreted by the thyroid gland that helps regulate body growth, development, and metabolic rate.

tincture: a solution of soluble plant constituents in a solvent menstruum. "Can you find the echinacea tincture? I feel a cold coming on."

tincture press: A tincture press is composed of 2 parallel platens on a frame that is rigged with a hydraulic jack and a pan fitted with a drain hole and a hose. The macerating extract is poured into a pressing cloth inside the pan and the cloth is folded over the top of the mass of herb to prevent it from squeezing out the sides. Then the platens are jacked together, thereby efficiently forcing the liquid from the herb. The crude tincture then pours down the drain hose into a receiving vessel.

tinea: ringworm or other fungal infections of the skin.

tinnitus: a roaring, ringing, singing, tinkling, or tonal sound in the ears.

tonic: promoting restoration and invigoration of body fluids, membranes, muscles, glands, nerves, organs, or body systems.

tonify: to invigorate the body and the bodily organs, imparting healthy tension and elasticity to the tissues.

toxic: an agent that is overtly harmful to living things.

toxin: a poisonous substance contained in a plant. "Castor beans contain a lethal toxin."

ulcer or ulceration: gradual disintegration of mucous membrane or skin resulting in a lesion—an open, craterous sore.

umbel: a flower cluster, usually rounded, with all stems springing from the same hub (e.g. the flower of khella, an herb in the family *Apiaceae*).

uric acid: an end-product of protein metabolism; a waste product that must be excreted from the body through the urine or through the sweat; molecular formula $C_5H_4N_3O_3$.

urogenital: pertaining to the urinary tract and the genital organs.

urticaria: nettle rash or hives; an allergic skin disorder marked by the eruption of raised, reddened wheals accompanied by intense itching.

V: abbreviation for "volume."

varicose veins: swollen and dilated blood vessels, usually found on the legs.

vascular: of or relating to a vessel for the conveyance of liquids. In humans, the *vascular system* carries blood and lymph; in plants the *vascular bundles* carry sap.

vegetable glycerin: glycerin produced from vegetable oils and fats, (usually from coconuts), as opposed to glycerin produced from processing animal fat.

vegetative: the growth stage of a plant.

veno-occlusive disease: a potentially fatal condition wherein the small veins of the liver become obstructed.

vermifuge: serving to destroy or dispel parasitic worms.

viscosity: the quality or state of being viscous; the thickness of a liquid; "This cold honey demonstrates high viscosity, and I believe it is breaking my spoon."

vital force: a kind of cellular intelligence capable of orchestrating physiological functions.

vitiligo: a skin condition resulting in depigmented patches; piebald skin.

volatile oils: aromatic plant oils (terpene-rich compounds otherwise known as essential oils), which are readily vaporized at relatively low temperatures. Volatile oils can be preserved in dilute form in alcoholic tinctures, and can be concentrated through steam distillation (e.g. tea tree oil, peppermint oil).

volatilization: escape of essential oils from the herb or herbal product; vaporizing.

GLOSSARY

vortex: In blending fresh herbs in a blender, the preparation is said to "vortex" when the herb and liquid swirl around, forming a tiny whirlpool in the center of the swirling mass.

W: abbreviation for weight.

warfarin: a compound originally invented to be used as a rat poison, but is now used at low concentration as an anticoagulant in pharmaceutical drugs, such as Coumadin.

wash: a strong decoction or tea, usually cooled, which is applied to an injury, using a clean washcloth, which may be repeatedly wrung out and reapplied.

zeroing: prior to weighing, the adjustment of a scale to zero, thereby making certain that it is accurate. "Without first zeroing the gram scale, I can never be sure if my seeds are weighed out exactly."

References Consulted and Recommended

Bensky, Dan. 2004. *Chinese Herbal Medicine Materia Medica, 3rd Edition.* Eastland Press, 1308 pp.

Blumenthal, M., T. Hall, A. Goldburg, J. Grunwald, C. Riggins, and S. Ristor, editors. 1998. *The Complete German Commission E Monographs—Therapeutic Guide to Herbal Medicines.* Translation of: *Komission E.* Klein, S., translator. Austin: American Botanical Council, 685 pp.

Cech, R. 2015. *Strictly Medicinal® Seeds Catalog,* Williams (OR): Strictly Medicinal, LLC, 88 pp.

Cech, R. 2002. *Growing At-Risk Medicinal Herbs.* Williams (OR): Horizon Herbs, 315 pp.

Cook, E. and E. Martin. 1885. (Reprinted 1936.) *Remington's Practice of Pharmacy.* Easton (PA): The Mack Publishing Co., 1511 pp.

Dick, W. *Dick's Encyclopedia of Practical Receipts and Processes or "How they did it in the 1870s."* New York: Funk and Wagnalls, 607 pp.

Felter, H. 1922. (Reprinted 1985.) *The Eclectic Materia Medica, Pharmacology and Therapeutics.* Portland (OR): Eclectic Medical Publishing. Vol. 1, 743 pp.

Felter, H. and J. Lloyd. 1898. (Reprinted: 1984.) *King's American Dispensatory*, Portland (OR): Eclectic Medical Publishing, Vol. 1 & 2, 2172 pp.

Foster, S. and J. Duke. 1977. *A Field Guide to Medicinal Plants: Eastern and North America.* Boston (MA): Houghton Mifflin Co., 341 pp.

Foster, S. and Yue Chongxi. 1992. *Herbal Emissaries.* Rochester, (VT): Healing Arts Press, 356 pp.

Grieve, M. 1931. *A Modern Herbal.* New York: Hafner Publishing Company Inc., Vol. 1 & 2, 866 pp.

Kapoor, L. 1990. *Handbook of Ayurvedic Medicinal Plants.* Boca Raton (FL): CRC press, 416 pp.

McGuffin, M., C. Hobbs, R. Upton, A. Goldburg. 1997. *Botanical Safety Handbook.* Boca Raton (FL): CRC press, 231 pp.

Moerman, D. 1986. *Medicinal Plants of Native America*, Ann Arbor (MI): University of Michigan Museum of Anthropology, Vol. 1, 534 pp.

Moore, M. 1979. *Medicinal Plants of the Mountain West*. Santa Fe, (NM): The Museum of New Mexico Press, 200 pp.

Moore, M. 1993. *Medicinal Plants of the Pacific West*. Santa Fe (NM): Red Crane Books, 359 pp.

Pharmacopoeia of the United States of America. 1955, 15th Revision. Easton (PA): Mack Publishing Co., 1178 pp.

Priest, A. and L. Priest. 1982. *Herbal Medication, a Clinical and Dispensary Handbook.* London: L.N. Fowler & Co. Ltd.,174 pp.

Theiss B. and P. Theiss. 1989. *The Family Herbal*. Rochester (VT): Healing Arts Press, 281 pp.

Tilford, Gregory. 1998. *From Earth to Herbalist*. Missoula (MT): Mountain Press Publishing Co., 249 pp.

Uphof, J. 1968. *Dictionary of Economic Plants.* New York: Stechert-Hafner Service Agency Inc., 591 pp.

Van Wyk, B., B. Van Oudtshoorn, and N. Gericke. 1997. *Medicinal Plants of South Africa.* Pretoria: Briza Publications, 304 pp.

Weiss, R. 1998, 6th ed. *Herbal Medicine*. Translation of: *Lehrbuch der Phytotherapie*. A. Meuss, translator. Beaconsfield: Beaconsfield Publishing, 362 pp.

Wichtl, M. and N. Bisset, editors. 1944. *Herbal Drugs and Phytopharmaceuticals*. Stuttgart: Medpharm Science, 566 pp.

Windholz, M., S. Budavari, R. Blumetti, and E. Otterbein, editors. 1983. *The Merck Index*. Rathway (NJ): Merck and Co. Inc., 1463 pp.

Plant Index

315

General Index

abrasions, 83, 140,

absolute alcohol content of spirits (formulas), 32–34

absolute alcohol content, tincture (formula), 38

absolute alcohol content of fresh herb tinctures with menstruum containing only alcohol, 37–8

absolute alcohol content of fresh herb tinctures with menstruum containing alcohol & water, 42

absolute alcohol content of dry herb tinctures, 38, 42, 44

absolute glycerin content, 60–2

absolute glycerin content (formula), 62

aceta (defined), 54

aceta (formula), 55

aceta, dry herb (procedure), 55

acetous tinctures (defined), 53

acetous tinctures (formula), 56

acetous tinctures (procedure), 56

acetous tinctures, low-dose (formula), 57

acetous tincures, low-dose (procedure), 57

aches & pains, 48, 98, 99, 101–2, 109, 124, 127, 131, 133, 136, 192, 220, 225, 240, 247, 260, 283, 286, 290-1, 293, 297

acid reflux, 106

acne, pimples & pustules, 29, 75, 101, 106, 118, 130, 135, 148, 151, 167, 235, 242, 272, 276, 289, 296-7

adaptogenic herbs, 48, 118–9, 171, 180–1, 205–7, 270–1, 280–1. 251–2, 270–1, 280–1

addiction, 133, 139, 215, 233, 293

adrenal burnout, 70, 118–9, 162, 215–6, 233

adverse reactions (explained), 51–2

alcohol (defined), 31

alcohol, diluted (formula), 33

alcohol, grain, 31–2

alcohol, organically certified, 32

alcohol:water ratio (defined), 31

alcoholism, 60, 278

alkalinizing herbs (high in chlorophyll), 148

alkaloidal salts (defined), 53–4

alkaloids (defined), 46

alkaloids, solubility, 39, 46

allergic responses to herbs (explained), 51

allergies, 76–7, 127, 199, 223, 231, 262

alterative herbs, 77, 143, 242–3, 244–6, 250–1

altitude sickness, 237, 252

analgesic herbs (see aches & pains)

anemia (see iron-building herbs)

anesthetic herbs, 121

antibacterial herbs (internal use), 72, 117, 123, 144, 163, 164–6, 168–70, 172, 177–8, 181, 182–4, 184–6, 191–3, 198–9, 201–2, 209–10, 220–1, 234, 235–6, 236–7, 256–7, 268–70, 270–1, 271–2, 276, 279, 283–4

anticancer herbs (see cancer)

antidepressant herbs, 124, 133, 138, 175, 212, 225–6, 248, 251–2, 255, 259–61

antiflatulent herbs (see carminative)

antifungal herbs, 106, 127, 128, 234, 256–7, 276, 280–1

anti-inflammatory herbs, 47, 85, 106, 109, 111, 112, 127, 133, 140, 162, 163, 165, 173, 175, 175–6, 186–7, 191–3, 203–5, 215–6, 224–5, 225–6, 244, 265–7, 270–1, 289, 290-1, 292, 297–8

327